I THINK
I LIKE
GIRLS

ROSIE DAY

I THINK I LIKE GIRLS

DISCOVERING YOUR SEXUAL IDENTITY

PIATKUS

PIATKUS

First published in Great Britain in 2025 by Piatkus

10 9 8 7 6 5 4 3 2 1

A CIP catalogue record for this book is available from the British Library.

ISBN 978-034944-200-6

Printed and bound in Great Britain by

Clays Ltd, Elcograf S.p.A.

Papers used by Piatkus are from well-managed forests and other responsible sources.

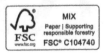

Some names and identifying characteristics have been changed to protect the privacy of the individuals involved.

Piatkus
An imprint of
Little, Brown Book Group
Carmelite House
50 Victoria Embankment
London EC4Y 0DZ

The authorised representative
in the EEA is
Hachette Ireland
8 Castlecourt Centre
Dublin 15, D15 XTP3, Ireland
(email: info@hbgi.ie)

An Hachette UK Company
www.hachette.co.uk

*To all the women who showed me
what was possible.*

Contents

Introduction   ix

Part One: Ready?

1   The first thought   3
2   I've got a girl crush   15
3   Hot takes history   29
4   Deconstruction of a lesbian   39

Part Two: Sex?

5   What's in a name?   49
6   H is for homophobe   59
7   I can't think straight   71
8   13 Going on 30   79
9   It's time to choose you   87
10   Throwing out your closet   97

Part Three: Go!

11   Lesbihonest   119
12   What is love?   141
13   Lez get together   145
14   Scissor sisters   157
15   Why don't you just leave?   179
16   How to heal from heartbreak   195
17   Lesbi long term   207
18   The kids are alright   215
19   What have you done today to make you feel proud?   227

Epilogue   235
Acknowledgements   237

Introduction

Before I embark on anything in life, I like to think 'Is this something that would have got me institutionalised in the nineteenth century?' – and if the answer is yes, then I'm on the right track. *Liking girls* is one of those acts.

That's easy for me to say now, but when it came to my sexuality that wasn't always the case. I spent twenty-five years in a closet so deep that the Pevensie children (of Narnia fame) were never going to find me, even with the help of a hot, sexy lion. Fresh out of a toxic relationship with a man, I had no idea how to tackle the one thing I knew I wanted: to date women.

The phrase 'I think I like girls' echoed in my brain as I floated down supermarket aisles. I thought about it while I sat at brunches with friends who spoke in depth about their latest crushes and boyfriends, while I stuffed avocado in my mouth to avoid answering questions about my love life. I was desperate for someone to talk to about it. Heck, I was desperate to watch something about it. The only film I'd seen was that French one that was so graphic my friend and I rolled out of the cinema giggling to disdainful looks and tuts from serious, art house film critics. Dating a woman seemed as impossible as winning the lottery. How would I even go about it? What was the difference between dating men and women? What does a same-sex relationship look like? What would people think? These were questions that regularly circled my brain late at night as I counted the cracks in my ceiling (twenty-three, plus two spiders and four cobwebs).

I was utterly confused and totally overwhelmed. I longed to be a kid again. At twelve I thought I knew everything. At twenty-five I felt I knew nothing. Twelve-year-old me didn't want anyone to tell her what to do, but me as an adult wanted to be told exactly what to do all the time and to just be given a wonderful girlfriend without ever having to put myself out there. Almost like those creepy men who order blow-up girlfriends off the internet . . . but less creepy. I had standards. I wanted mine to be alive.

Growing up I never really gave my sexual identity much thought. I lived in the suburbs, in one of those beige towns that suck the life right out of you. The sort of place where you feel claustrophobic outside. We moved constantly, my life measured in duct tape and sore fingers from folding thick cardboard as we piled our identities again and again into the back of removal vans – a piece of me getting lost along each A road. I was too busy trying to design my perfect bedroom (only for it to be ripped away from me a few months later) to give my sexuality too much thought.

In Hampshire, amongst the skin-tight, see-through leggings and Ugg boots, bluetoothing songs to one another as we crowded on the school steps at lunch time, being gay was never discussed. Unless it was a slur thrown by a boy with too much hair gel, his spikes about as dangerous as a hedgehog's. Girls whispered about who'd done what with who. Who was making out on the school playing field. Who slept together at the party last Friday night. And I pretended to get excited. I could feign delight and giggles over the latest salacious comment, and 'ooo' at the correct times. I didn't care much for people my own age. I didn't want to be there. I knew I was desperate to escape the humdrum afternoons of rounders and ballet. I knew there was so much more to life and I was a whippet pounding against the gate, ready to sprint the moment I got the chance. I suspected I was different. A lifetime of being a child actor had meant I was adept at flitting between personalities and groups of people. I knew I could be many things – but it never crossed my mind that I might be gay.

My first relationships were with men, because I was trying to conform to societal expectations. But when I landed in my twenties I couldn't deny the thought that kept crossing my mind. Underneath the faux heterosexuality, and the combined pressures of feeling I had to find a husband, a white picket fence (rented obvs – no one in my generation is buying a house), and 2.5 children by thirty (let me skip to the part where I tell you I've failed at all of those), I was secretly watching videos of Emily Blunt under my duvet. 'Good girl' conditioning had sent a clear message to me: don't be too much and don't want too much. Live the life society expects of you. Don't rock the boat. When you've been walking a particular path for so long it can seem impossible, or even dangerous, to veer off it.

Until the 'I can't do it any more' moment, a moment which is almost certainly always shouted by a girl who's not only going to do it, but do it well.

Our brains are wired to choose familiar hell over unfamiliar heaven, so it was inevitable that it was going to be a bit of a ride to get me to live authentically. What followed was a journey of exploration, reflection, doing 'the work' (which is therapy speak for dealing with your shit), and watching lots of TikToks of Margot Robbie.

In a world where most females are subconsciously looking for safety, it makes sense that doing anything that puts your head above the parapet can seem dangerous to some aspect of ourselves. It's scary, especially for those who are not modelled authenticity or healthy relationships growing up. There can be a ton of shame, embarrassment and fear of the unknown. This is a process of learning who we really are, what we want and how to get there. We have to shed the negative conditioning that we've absorbed from society, our surroundings and at times from family members. If there's a little voice inside you that's telling you that exploring your sexuality isn't OK, you need to know that someone put that voice there. It's not yours.

Just a heads-up that feelings are a key part of this process – and few of us get taught how to sit with our feelings. But instead of burying or ignoring them, you can see them as information. Feelings tell us what's right or wrong for us, what to move towards (Taylor Swift) and what to run away from (Donald Trump). They need to be met with curiosity: and the good thing is that this kind will not kill your cats (trust me, I have a lot of cats and a lot of feelings, and no one's died just yet).

You might be coming to this book at the very start of your exploration into your sexuality; maybe you've seen the title and recognised that you too have that thought. Or maybe you're well on the Rainbow Brick Road. We're going to cover everything from first feelings to marriage and kids, and a lot in between. Feel free to skip around to what's relevant to you. There are subjects within these pages that may bring up heavy emotions for you: abusive relationships, sexual assault and eating disorders. I don't want to shy away from the truth that women today live with, but I do promise you that this book is one of hope.

Now, as the great Maya Angelou says, 'A bird doesn't sing because it has an answer, it sings because it has a song' – I don't have all the answers. I like to think that this isn't a case of the blind leading the blind, but more that you're driving the car and I'm alongside you making sure we don't career into a quarry. Hopefully there's a hot girl for you to date at the end of this road trip and, if not, you'll continue your exploration into who you are while singing '9 to 5' on repeat. Your sexuality is a part of that. And it's your birthright to explore it.

My life is infinitely better for being free, for being able to discover new things about myself and for living authentically. As I always say, 'Do it for the plot'! And what is personal is often universal, and my journey may resonate with someone else.

When I speak of girls and women within this book, I want to make it clear that this is for anyone who identifies as such, including readers who may be non-binary. While my experience is from a gender-conforming perspective, *everyone is welcome here.*

This book is not Lesbian 101 (but I defo would have taken that class if it had been offered to me). It's more of a helping hand, sharing everything I've learnt and been taught by the women who came before me. I can't give all the answers, or answers that are necessarily the right ones for you. But I can share my path and my perspective, and hopefully I can be alongside you in this journey as a fellow traveller.

So if like me, you like to pretend your life's a movie, turn the page and whisper:

I'm ready for a new story to begin.

PART ONE

READY?

The first thought

Dear Diary,

I'm splayed out in the bathtub akin to Ophelia in the lake but moderately less dead. I say moderately because I've just been steamrolled by the news my ex was cheating on me.

I count the cracks in the bathroom tiles, listening to the monotonous drip-drip from the tap. I know the journey ahead of me looms large, and I'm at the bottom of a colossal mountain of healing, but there's a lightness to my body I haven't had in years. Or maybe I've put too many Epsom salts in the water again.

'I'm free,' I whisper with absolutely no irony, as if I'm in some quirky A24 coming of age movie. It's 3 p.m. and I'm picking dry Cheerios out of a bowl I've managed to float on the surface of the water. Classic 'my life's imploded' behaviour.

The truth that I've admitted to no one is: I was scared I was going to have to marry that man. But more than that, I was scared I was going to have to marry any man – because I was going to die having never explored the truth: that I like girls.

Whatever happens now, I'm not going back. This is it. The dark steps leading up to the murky attic where Dorian Gray's painting *sits have collapsed under the weight of deep truths and years of denial. (I'm hoping there are some girls up there too.)*

If there was a camera focusing on me in this moment, I'd peer over the bathtub and look straight down the lens, asking: 'Now how the hell do I do this?'

Love,

Rosie x

The realisation started with a bleach-blonde theatre director who kept fondly referring to me as a dick. 'What are you doing, you dick? You're meant to be on the other side of the stage.' Usually someone talking to me like that would send me into a spiral of anxiety and self-criticism, but there was something about the tone of her words that felt electric.

Soon I was arriving at rehearsals early for coffee, buoyed by the promise of a simple conversation. I was hitting my marks perfectly, I was practising my best witty comebacks and remarkably I found a song named after her by Girl In Red (who I would later learn is a lesbian icon) that I could pour out my feelings to on the last Tube home. What was this feeling I was having? Why did I want to be near her all the time? Why did it feel like there were a million butterflies in my chest when she was around? I'd sit in a nearby café playing over our interactions, confused by what was happening. I'd only dated boys up until this point and was nervous of this newfound feeling of excitement laced with fear.

I'd suspected for a few years that maybe I was into girls, but I'd always suppressed the thought as quickly as it entered my mind. As they say, denial is a river in Egypt and I was the captain of the local ferry service. I barely knew anyone who was dating a woman. Sex education at school was purely heterosexual, and growing up I didn't even know a lesbian – down in the paper towns of Hampshire they were about as common as unicorns.

It wasn't until my twenty-second birthday party in a wanky bar in Soho – the sort where cocktails are served in paint pots and they're playing 'beats' that disguise themselves as music – that my friend, Jess, arrived wearing a very unusual fedora. As we sat curled up on the sofa where I'd thrown myself at her, she promptly told me she was dating a girl. I swear, magical, twinkling princess music played as if a fairy godmother had waved a magic wand. The perfect birthday present. Finally, SOMEONE I could talk to about the things I thought about late at night (not like that . . . ! OK, maybe a little). Never had I been so invested in a friend's relationship. I wanted updates, and I wanted to understand what it was like to date a girl. I wanted to be Jess, but I wasn't sure I could do it for myself. Jess had a level of self-assurance I could only dream of, not only in her excellent choice of headwear but also the way she moved through the world so freely.

The thought of dating a girl kept cropping up like whack-a-mole – no matter how hard I smacked it away, it kept coming back. I know now that if you suppress the truth that you do know about yourself, you're never going to be satisfied. Accepting what you know is the first step to accepting yourself. And if you're thinking that you think you might like girls, the chances are you do. Psychologist Carl Rogers once said, 'The curious paradox is that when I accept myself exactly as I am, then I can change.' Once you begin to accept your sexuality, the exploration can begin.

A journey of sexual exploration

My exploration began when I was working in Europe. On my first night, still covered in plane sweat, I was trying to persuade my key card to let me into my hotel room (is there anything more annoying than having to traipse back down to reception when it doesn't work?). A gentle voice interrupted my wrestling match with the door handle, 'You're Rosie, aren't you?' And I spun around to be met by one of the most beautiful people I'd ever seen.

My new co-worker and I went for dinner, and by the end of the night we were both convinced we'd met our soulmate. I spent three months joined at the hip with a girl I adored, in one of the most fun cities in the world. And then, as quickly as it had started, the job ended. I went back to England and she flew back over the Atlantic Ocean. And a few months later . . . I was dating a man.

I was knuckling down on being straight, while being perplexed by my identity. And figuring out your identity as a whole is a bigger question we'll come to later. Exploring where you sit in the world and where you want to be are two huge questions that often send me into an existential crisis. We are constantly being told how we should act, what we should have and who we should be – so how are we even supposed to get to know OURSELVES? If, like me, your brain is 80 per cent TikTok trends, 10 per cent iced lattes and 10 per cent the whereabouts of Taylor Swift, you don't have time to find out who you are.

But we do. We all have time. We just live in a society that functions better when we're all dissociated and not prioritising our well-being.

The first thing to know about sexuality is that for many it's something that's fluid. We're not bound to whatever we choose on a random Wednesday in June. It doesn't have to stay the same. Sexuality is a spectrum and everyone's on it. While some people might think their history of past relationships accurately reflects their sexuality, for many that's not the case. Your relationship history doesn't determine your sexual orientation: you do. It is completely possible to consider whether your sexuality may have changed and to explore it – or maybe it's something you've always known and you're ready to step out into the sun.

After all, attraction is supposed to feel good. If being in relationships with men isn't appealing to you, or if you can't truly see yourself ending up happy, or if your attraction to men makes you uncomfortable, it's a sure-fire sign that you may be looking at the wrong sex.

So, you might be giving penises the chop? (Ouch, but lol.) You are Princess Anne riding to King Charles's coronation like she's ready to take down Napoleon? (After that kickass display, I'm sort of hoping Anne hops over to the LGBTQIA+ community with that fabulous cape.) You're feeling like William the Conqueror, ready to explore a land filled with pussy . . . cats (get your head out of the gutter)? But how exactly do you explore your sexuality?

Like anything important, start slow. You don't have to jump into bed with that hot person who sits next to you at work or hook up with the girl you smiled at on the Tube. Like getting into a pool, you sometimes have to dip your toe in first instead of diving right in so you don't get such a shock you have to be pulled out by the lifeguard. (Me, swimming, every summer.)

In my experience, the most important relationship you have to have first is with yourself. Acceptance and appreciation for what you like (or think you might like) and being comfortable with who you are come first and that can take a long time to build. As my therapist says, 'Baby steps, they really add up.'

Know what you know. Don't lie to yourself. It's amazing what we can hide from our own selves. Turns out I like cucumber (who knew) and for my entire life I thought I hated it. And turns out I like girls.

So welcome back to school, but with fewer thirteen-year-old boys shouting out comments in the classroom. You might be wondering how come it's taken you this long to pick up this book? How come it's taken me this long to write this book? I'd like to introduce a term that provides the answer to both those questions: compulsory heterosexuality. God – it sounds as depressing as compulsory PE.

We are not all straight by default

Compulsory heterosexuality is exactly what it says on the tin. Being straight is something that society tries to force on us, like your mum trying to make you eat broccoli or your boss demanding that you work from the office every day of the week. Compulsory heterosexuality is the assumption that we are all straight by default. From the day we come out looking like little jacket potatoes, we're trained to think we will find someone of the opposite gender to mate with. From a biological standpoint of continuing the human race it makes sense, but there's more to it than that. It's a trap. Compulsory heterosexuality ties in with the misogyny that causes women's sexualities and lives to be defined by men. When a friend goes through a break-up and we hear the all-familiar, 'But I don't know who I am without him', this is because since day dot we've been conditioned to believe that we are defined by a relationship with a man. It makes sense when throughout history we were literally sold by our fathers like monopoly houses to the highest bidder.

So where is the boundary between our own thoughts and what society has imposed on us? From birth we're constantly picking up cues on what is acceptable and what is not. We subconsciously monitor our environment and the behaviour of others to keep ourselves safe. From when we're little we're generally taught 'it's wrong to steal', 'it's good to pay taxes', 'girls are meant to fall in love with boys' – so what happens when we have a thought that pushes back on those beliefs? Do we end up as a tax-avoiding lesbian with an amazing array of Gucci handbags? (Yes . . .) Or do we end up with some sort of inner turmoil? For me it was the latter. I had to separate my thoughts into laundry bins, the colours and the darks and the whites. What had been given to me by my parents, my environment and my friends, and what really was mine: what I wanted and who I was.

My life was a whole load of 'I should', 'I shouldn't', 'I must', 'I have to' and not a lot of 'Who the fuck am I and what do I want?' As young women, we often feel everyone else knows more than us. There's some encyclopaedia of 'knowing best' and it's already been checked out of the library. It's easy to get swept away and follow along. But you have an inner knowing that needs to be tapped into. We're all born with an innate knowing of ourselves, the lights that slowly get switched off and disconnected through experiences and by people. Amongst the clutter of self-criticism, TikTok trends and useless facts there's a source inside your body that knows what's right for you. It's like having a hundred tabs open on your laptop and eventually finding the ASOS sale one. You just have to reconnect. Listening to yourself or 'listening within' means tuning in to how you're feeling, what you're thinking, and what you need.

The first thing we need to do is observe ourselves. We need to zoom in deep inside (like birdwatchers but sexier) and witness our thoughts and feelings. Pah! you might think, I know everything there is to know about me! I thought the same . . . turns out I knew everything about the version of me I'd created to appease others and how I operated in the world, and very little of myself internally. Maybe I just didn't want to look, because I didn't want to have to go there. Bit like a smear test, put it off until your life is actually under threat (I'm kidding, ladies, don't be doing that). But connecting with our inner world and what we really think is key to getting to know our sexuality. How often have you agreed with someone in a conversation and then later thought, 'Hang on, I didn't mean that'? Or not realised how you felt about a comment until it's too late to say something? So many of us are disconnected and distracted by the grind of the everyday to stop and look inward. It's like stopping to smell the flowers, when the flowers are powerful home truths that might make you cry.

So here are five quick questions to kick off the road to exploration:

1   Are your feelings towards men and women different? If so, how are they different?

2   When your straight friends talk about the people they fancy, do you relate to them?

3   When you dream or fantasise about a partner, who are you imagining?

4   Do you feel like you could live with a woman in a romantic way, even if you can't imagine doing anything sexual with a woman?

5   Can you picture yourself dating, loving, having sex with or marrying a woman?

For transparency, here are my answers. However, these are not the answers I would have given at the start of this journey:

1   I feel safe and held around most women. When it comes to men I'm happy to hang out with them, but I don't want them in my house and meeting my cats.

2   I can totally appreciate the hot men my friends are into. I have eyes. I've watched Ryan Gosling perform 'I'm Just Ken' maybe five thousand times. I just don't think I want them in my bed.

3   When I dream about a partner, it's a hot slightly older woman with a kickass career and excellent taste in interior design.

4   Yes, I have a fantasy about living in a beautiful old cottage with a garden adorned with roses and puddleducks where we bake banana bread and read Jane Austen together.

5   Yes, yes, yes and yes.

If your answers to the questions lead to the statement or realisation of 'I think I like girls', then please read on. And even if you're just a bit curious, stick around: it's going to be girl-orious.

At first I was certain I wasn't gay because I wasn't sure I wouldn't change my mind (I haven't, but it was greeeaaatt to have that anxiety). Worrying that you can't be 100 per cent certain does not mean you can't be gay. In life we want things to be binary – black or white, yes or no – but sexuality is a spectrum. There's no percentage-based test you need to pass. I felt like I almost needed to prove I was gay, like I had a driving licence to whack out whenever somebody asked about my sexuality. You can identify as gay if you've liked men in the past but are no longer attracted to men or want to pursue relationships with them. Many girls who identify as queer have dated or had genuine relationships with men before coming to the realisation they weren't straight. That doesn't make them any less of a lesbian. The maths isn't in our favour: it can take a long time to figure out you're gay. The whole 'If you're a girl you're supposed to like boys' thing, and going through the process of discovering yourself and what you like, is an entire movie plot you have to tread through. And statistically only 6 per cent of the population is gay so it takes a while to find people.

But what it didn't take me long to find were the patterns lining up like rows on Grandma's jumper, and there was one I could not deny: my girl crushes.

2

I've got a girl crush

Dear Diary,

My first girl crush at school was a sixth former named Alex. I'd found myself at an all-girls' secondary school with bright purple blazers that kids from the local comprehensive threw pens at when we got off the bus. One night they chased eleven-year-old me through the woods. Year 7 felt as grown-up an age one could be: pink Motorola flip phone, heeled shoes and a weekly fiver to buy treats from the corner shop. As someone who'd survived the worst of school dinners, I felt like I'd landed on my feet. I should mention that prior to this, aged nine, I had a thing with Sandra Bullock in a Holiday Inn on the outskirts of Leeds. And by 'thing' I mean I watched the VHS tape of Miss Congeniality *under the scratchy hotel bed sheets and had an experience I didn't understand.*

Alex was eighteen, blonde and the definition of high school hot. Oh, and the leader of the school drama club. Why an all-girls' school was performing Nicholas Nickleby *is beyond me, but I didn't care – we got two rehearsals a week after school and that meant more time for me to bask in her presence. There were three Year 7s all obsessed with her. We formed a gang (if a gang meant giving her notes written in glittery gel pens and hugs every time we saw her, and the gang members could only take out your kneecaps). We left her voicemails. Once we even dug out the Yellow Pages to find her home address, ringing all the numbers listed to try and track her down – what can I say, we were smitten. Cut to ten years later and she's performing in a local theatre production of Shakespeare's* All's Well That Ends Well. *I'm in my twenties, having returned home to see my sister, when Alex strides out on stage. She is exactly as I remember her, only now she is alarmingly . . . normal? The girl I painted as my hero is lovely. But she's not the goddess I'd imagined her when I was eleven.*

Crushes are just that: crushes. They're small phases of obsession that give us a bit of a buzz and make life a little brighter. They can feel like everything, and then a few months later, nothing at all.

When Alex left for university I was crushed. I was devastated to the point that I wrote her a song. I was tempted to write the lyrics in this book, but for eleven-year-old Rosie's dignity I'll refrain. And then I recorded it in my weekly guitar lesson. Burnt it on to a CD and gave it to her. Everyone heard said song and didn't put two and two together that they might be harbouring a soon-to-be homosexual. But like most things in my family, no one batted an eyelid. (If anyone has a copy, please burn it.)

Love,
Rosie x

As the band Little Big Town once sang in dulcet country tones, 'I've got a girl crushhhh.' While I was hopeful it was going to be a wonderful anthem for gay girls to sing loudly in the bathroom mirror while using a toothbrush as a microphone and strumming the belly of a very belligerent cat as a guitar (just me?), it turned out to be a song about a woman who had a crush on a girl purely because that girl was in a relationship with the guy she fancied, and she just wanted to be her so she could get off with him. Like a queer-baiting version of 'Girlfriend' by Avril Lavigne, but much sexier.

God damn it. Where are the excellent lesbian anthems, please?

But back to the point: GIRL CRUSHES. We've all been there, and we've all got one (don't deny it). Even most straight women have another woman on their hall pass. We have the traditional categories: celebrity girl crushes (hello, Margot Robbie, Beyoncé, Jennifer Aniston); workplace crushes on older, wiser, hotter bosses (looking at you, *The Devil Wears Prada*); movie crushes (Gemma Arterton in *St Trinian's* is canon for most gay girlies); and then there's the schoolgirl crushes on the girl two years above or the new PE teacher that gives you attention. Looking back, I can give multiple examples of all four, which probably should have been a rainbow warning flag, but society kept me more strait-laced than a whalebone corset.

But then there are the more (potentially) realistic crushes. A new friend who makes you laugh more than you have in ages, and you find yourself always wanting to hang out with her. An old friend who always makes slight sexual innuendoes, with whom you have great banter. Someone you can't wait to text back, who makes your heart skip when they hug you. Have you got a 'girl crush'? Or a real crush? How do you know? A good question to ask is . . . do you want to BE them, or do you want to be WITH them?

We're so often enamoured by a hot, powerful woman who looks like they have it all, that there's a part within ourselves that wants to emulate them. After all, if women were taught compassion for themselves, the economy would collapse! Maybe we desire their style, their friends, their power, their lives. So, is that what you're feeling? Or do you see a world in which a relationship is possible? We're so used to perfect, airbrushed pictures online that when we see women who appear totally unaffected and who share their seemingly normal (but still aspirational) lives, we often become infatuated with their genuine outlook on life. I fully believe we should have people we admire, look up to and inspire us to be better: our 'North Star' as the American motivational speaker Mel Robbins calls it (hers is Dwayne Johnson, aka The Rock!). It's easy to confuse that infatuation with a real desire to be in relationship when you're opening yourself up to your sexuality. I want a great girlfriend *and* a great coat!

Do I love her or am I *in love* with her?

It's normal to find yourself feeling emotionally and physically comfortable with a close friend, so this doesn't necessarily mean that you want to take the relationship further either physically or romantically. But sometimes it does, and if that's the case, a conversation could be had with them. If you're finding it hard to know whether it's friendship or romance, wanting to spend as much time together as possible is a pretty good indicator of romantic feelings. Preferring to be alone with them instead of in a group is an even stronger sign.

Think about why you'd like to take this relationship to the next stage. What makes you think that the two of you would be good together? Is there potential for longevity, or are you risking a friendship for a fling? If you're sure about it can you bring the subject up? Sometimes all you need is two minutes of insane courage to change your life. If you feel too nervous to do it in person, maybe write down your thoughts and feelings in a text or seven-minute voice note they can listen to on 1.5x speed. You can tell them that if it's not reciprocated that's totally OK, and you don't want it to affect your already sterling friendship. As the saying goes, nothing ventured, nothing gained! I know the prospect of making things awkward between the two of you is terrifying, but if it's someone you feel close to chances are they'll be glad you trusted and valued them enough to tell them.

And if we're treating our initial experiences like an exercise to explore this side of ourselves, it's OK if it doesn't always go to plan! You're a scientist conducting research! It's possible you're going to have an experience with a girl and feel unsure, or it might be a light-bulb moment and you're certain it's what you want. It's different for everyone. And when the elders in your life may say, 'Are you sure?' you're allowed to answer, 'I don't know. I'm still figuring this out.'

I once fell for one of my friends and it went like this:

Portobello Road. Notting Hill. The backdrop to one of the greatest love stories of all time. A floppy-haired Hugh Grant strolls through the markets and the seasons change as he pines for the hottest thing on earth: nineties' Julia

Roberts. During the five million times that I watched that film, never did I think I would find myself at the centre of my very own W11 love story.

Everyone's having their Saturdays in individual bubbles. Their own dramas playing out over brunch that I'm not privy to. Above the hustle and bustle of the market stalls and crowded streets, 15 feet up, we lie on a balcony, glazing ourselves in body oil. Tourists pass, shouting up to us, their words barely reaching us before being swallowed up by a symphony of Taylor Swift. We feel a tinge of smugness when we gaze down at the chaos below. How did we end up here on this glorious sunny Saturday? Bella decamped from America - partly for university that turned into a full-time job, partly to escape from her home life. Her flat becomes a place of solace from a scrapbook millennial life.

We bask in the sun, talking therapy, the Eras tour, the state of the government and the many dates she's been on with various guys that we dissect like neurosurgeons. We sit in shorts and bikinis listening to Lana Del Rey. I'm living the A24 movie, guys. But Bella isn't looking at me.

She's obsessing over a guy named Paul, who on the scale of humanity is a solid three. Bella is a ten.

One weekend we spend an entire day planning how to casually drop into a party that we know Paul will be at. We even rope in my friend Ruby as someone who is throwing the 'other party we have to go to' to look like Bella's in demand. We put so much brain power into this evening, I thought I was going to be meeting the Duke of Hastings from *Bridgerton*. And when Paul walks in, I almost burst out laughing. He speaks with a lispy voice and tells us he'd been playing *FIFA* indoors – on one of the hottest days of the year. My stomach sinks as I realise that yet another of my friends is falling over themselves to be with a guy who would be so lucky to date them.

Girls so often don't realise the power we have because society doesn't want us to have it. Girls are squashed. We make ourselves small, both metaphorically and literally. We don't want to take up space in case our thoughts and ideas are too much. Heaven forbid we make someone else uncomfortable by being ourselves. I'm reminded of the fact that 'if that makes sense' is only ever said by girls who have never not made sense of their lives. A conditioning of self-doubt and good girl livelihoods. And now Bella is objectively settling for someone who has the personality of a Great Dane.

The night I met Bella my Pisces horoscope told me I was going to meet the love of my life. This I knew in hindsight, reading it just before I went to bed. I read horoscopes at the end of the day lest they influence the pathway of my day. At a summer party at a house in Hampstead that came complete with pizza chef and wood-fired oven, I walked in to see a girl clad in cowboy boots chatting away. I barely had time to put down the cheap potted plant I'd brought before I was swept into a conversation with her. As someone who has the attention span of a rogue four-year-old – I was laser-focused all night. She agrees. It was like there was no one else in the room. I saw our mutual friend laughing behind her as we talked. When I investigated later, my friend said she thought Bella liked guys and maybe girls, but wasn't sure.

So instead we stick to friendship. The world reveals itself to us in such similar ways that we finish each other's sentences. Moments spent cycling around London seem so precious that I think we need a Beatles soundtrack to blare out around us. I wait for one of us to get hit off our bike. I wait for it to end. It doesn't. She reads books so old they're tainted by time and the Sunday papers and laughs at the political columns I can't understand. Her red Roberts radio plays the soundtrack to our summer. Shading her face in her blue baseball cap, her freshly painted burgundy nails bleeding onto the page, she is effortlessly stylish.

We plan a summer holiday to Ischia. We'll stay at an Italian monastery cut off by the rolling tide twice a day that looks over a water-coloured town of fishing boats and pebbled beaches.

I can see it in my mind's eye, we're reading Deborah Levy in crumpled linen shirts over our matching floral bikinis, our hair curled from the sea water, like something out of a rebranded H&M campaign.

And then I get a job doing a play and Bella has to work. Our summer melts away as we cancel our Booking.com reservation and prepare for the wettest (not like that) summer on record.

So instead we prepare for a summer of balcony days. We eat sourdough and cured meats and tiny tomatoes drizzled in olive oil from the deli on the corner.

Even on cloudy days the sun seems to permanently shine on this safe haven in central London. I watch the clouds weave their way around the sun. I keep staring at them to the point of blindness, trying to make sure I can watch which way they're headed. As if a single grey moment could taint this picture-perfect summer.

One evening I confide in my friend, who gives me some painfully obvious advice: 'You guys should get drunk on red wine and make out.'

Thanks for that – it hadn't occurred to me.

We had got drunk on a few occasions and one evening, after one glass too many of sparkling rosé, we ended up in the library of an old house, where Bella and I flopped on a shabby, dilapidated sofa. It was Christmas and the fire was roaring. Despite the muffled thuds of the party echoing through the walls, we felt separate from the rest. In this still, quiet moment, as the alcohol swam over us ... I couldn't do it. Dutch courage didn't give me enough courage. And then two bleary-eyed boys crashed in wanting to do coke off the fireplace. Vibe. Ruined. So I decide I'm OK in our chamber of friendship.

We stumble towards womanhood together. A prolonged adolescence feels necessary and we haven't passed out into weekly food shopping and mortgages. We pound the farmers' market each Sunday, spending our earnings on tulips and peonies, knowing we deserve to decorate our lives with blossoms.

We just sort of fit.

As she lies on the decking, I try to memorise everything about us.

The usual Sunday papers are laid out, pots of berries, it's so Instagrammable it makes me feel sick. We settle in to our weekend routine, soundtracked by HAIM and giggles and passages from our favourite books that sum up the very moment we're in. I wish I could read her this one:

'I'm in a holding pattern for a plane that may never take off.'

There's not much more to say, other than: it happens. The same way friends of the opposite sexes fall for each other – it happens with female friendships too. The only difference is we've been indoctrinated by excellent romcoms of guys and girls falling for their best friends, who are usually with somebody incredibly mean, or at the very least totally wrong for them, until they change their mind last minute (side note: did you know that if you object when the vicar asks 'Do you know of any reason why these two should not be wed,' even if you do it as a joke, the wedding can't go ahead, because they have to go all Miss Marple and investigate?). There's nothing wrong with falling for your friends. Life happens!

If you're coming to this later in life, have a think about how you were within relationships in your teenage years. Were there any feelings towards girls at that time? Growing up I never pursued people, I was just waiting for someone to come along and pursue me. I wasn't foaming at the mouth over the Jonas Brothers or desperate to sit next to a certain boy in maths class (unless I could copy his answers). If we had to pick a guy we fancied I would pull a random name out of thin air. I also definitely pretended I was 'dating' a boy at a local youth theatre. Plot twist: we both turned out to be gay.

Because I grew up very straight presenting, it was just assumed by my friends that men were going to come along at some point and maybe ask me out. At no point did I think, 'Who do I want to date?' At no point did anyone tell me I had the power to pursue whoever I wanted. It didn't even cross my mind. I thought men were the only option. And I was disappointed. A lot of women are used to the idea that men are supposed to be shit or underwhelming. We've normalised their bad behaviour to the point where it's basically accepted as par for the course. They are supposed to be annoying because they haven't interrogated their underlying misogyny.

I gaslit myself a lot because I thought I just had high standards for men, and I did away with any intrusive thoughts of women.

I also had really intense friendships with girls who were a bit older than me. The sort of ride-or-die, bury-the-body-in-the-backyard kind of friendships, waiting for them to text me back and getting a thrill when they did sort of friendships, which maybe should have been a clue. Wouldn't take Poirot to figure out what was going on. You can also still have crushes on male celebrities or characters from books and TV shows. I can still appreciate the other sex and it not determine my sexuality. It doesn't suddenly make you straight if you get a lot of shirtless Ryan Gosling videos popping up on your For You Page.

Looking back, there were definitely clues where my life was headed, but hindsight is 20:20. Consider the following clues, that may (or may not) resonate from your past:

- Being eager to impress specific women (but not men).
- Imagining what it might be like to kiss a particular girl.
- Loving storylines that feature LGBTQIA+ characters.
- Getting butterflies or feeling like you can't get close enough to a friend you really like.
- Experiencing strong feelings of admiration for a specific female teacher, actor or celebrity when you were growing up, that almost bordered on obsessive.
- Having an unusually close relationship with a female friend that was different and special in a way you couldn't articulate.
- Thinking relationships could be simpler: 'If only I were attracted to women/my best friend who would be perfect for me if she/I wasn't a girl.'
- Being in relationships with men and just not feeling that into it.

I so badly wanted to be in love with men. My brain had been consumed by every teenage book and movie out there. I was meant to have a Hilary Duff making out with Chad Michael Murray in the rain/Anne Hathaway's foot popping in *The Princess Diaries* moment. That's what young girls were told to aspire to. I hoped that my attraction to them would kick in eventually and I was just a late bloomer. Maybe when

I was fifty I'd wake up and be delivered a man I fancied by a nice stork?

Don't get me wrong, I loved my first boyfriend. He was the sweetest, and our relationship felt like the kind of first love described in young adult novels. But I loved him in the way I loved my chocolate Labrador. Very happy to cuddle and pat on the head, but I had to act my way through sexual attraction, like I'd seen in movies (with my boyfriend, not my dog, not that kind of book). I knew what to say, what to do, how to bite my lip (cringe) – essentially what I had been taught by society. There were times I would have done anything to be attracted to men so that I could fit neatly into the role that was expected of me, but I just couldn't. And I am such a people pleaser I would have done anything to make sure everyone else around me was comfortable with who I was. I didn't want to make myself smaller and not exist any more. I just couldn't make myself do it (no offence guys).

I dreaded my future with a man. After the image of a Disney-approved happily-ever-after had faded, the day-to-day idea of cohabiting with a man made me feel trapped. As iconic, gay pop star Chappell Roan says, the last thing you want to be doing is waking up married to a man, daydreaming about what life could have been like if you'd just given it a go with a woman. Sometimes it just takes a few seconds of bravery to change your life.

I just wanted to be 'normal'. (What even is that? There is literally no such thing.)

But in realising and accepting that I might be gay, that I didn't have a future with men, there was a sort of grief for the life that part of me had dreamed of. Society had sold me the dream of a perfect family with 2.4 children, a husband and a Toyota estate. Now the fantasy had to include a rich wife and a potentially better car. I knew that liking girls meant my life was going to be slightly less easy than I had imagined. I had always been strong and independent, but there was part of me that had fantasised a world where I cooked dinner while the children played in the garden and my (very rich) husband would burst through the door with a bunch of flowers and then we would all snuggle on the sofa together. Now I realise I need to be the very rich man of the family and my life is going to look a bit different from that. And as I've slowly learnt, seeing the world through a sapphic gaze is a pretty lovely way to view it versus a straight man's lens. I have realised that I'm able to appreciate so many things about myself and others, rather than focus on what men value in me (my face, my compliance). I notice women's tone of voice, their expressions, the specifics, all indicators to me that I am attracted to someone. I had been in a couple of relationships with men before but that didn't take away from my sexuality. Attraction is super-complicated. (There are people infatuated with the Golden Gate Bridge, don't forget!) It's possible to recognise a man *is* attractive but not be attracted *to* him. And once I got my head round the semantics of it all and the realisation that there are no rules . . . it was time to explore.

3

Hot takes history

Dear Diary,

My biggest achievement to date is that I didn't drop a single mark in my GCSE history paper. I am technically a historical genius. I am the David Attenborough of the Wars of the Roses (OK, maybe more Philomena Cunk). But I don't think lesbians were ever mentioned. Who am I kidding? Women barely got a look-in. Probably because they were too busy being locked up in corsets (it's no wonder they couldn't do much, when they literally couldn't breathe) and dying in childbirth trying to give their sour husbands a male heir so they didn't get beheaded.

And if women were around, they were usually to blame. It was all Henry doesn't like being married so he'll create a new religion to get out of it and Menelaus hates Helen even though he definitely started the war and if you choose to be single they'll call you a witch and drown you in the lake. I like to think they teach LGBTQIA+ history in schools now, but seeing as there's not enough money in all the world to get me to swing back through the gates of a school (though I would quite like to be the person to bring bunches back, Baby Spice style), it's more of a prayer than a fact. So . . . Who is the OG lesbian? Who's been paving the way before us? (I really hope it's

Joan of Arc. WHAT A BABE.) Where is our history and where do we come from?

Love,
Rosie x

We've got maybe four role models, we're not allowed on TV unless we're the gay best friend with one line, and Queen Victoria didn't believe we existed . . . The first time anyone has ever seen reality TV centred around lesbian relationships was in all likelihood recently when *I Kissed a Girl* dropped on iPlayer.

The question 'Where did lesbians originate?' sort of makes us sound like a very fine rare red wine (we totally are). But we weren't suddenly invented like an iPhone or Kim Kardashian's appearing and disappearing butt. We've been lesbianing (is it a verb? It is now!) throughout history.

The good news is since men all but erased us from history, while being gay in the UK was only legalised in 1967 for men, it's technically never been illegal for women, even though it was deeply frowned upon. When a law to criminalise homosexuality was proposed, it originally applied to both sexes, but Queen Victoria was of the opinion that such things would be a physical impossibility between women and no one had the guts to correct her – so the law was never passed. There have long been rumours of queens playing both sides, with one of the most popular originating in the early eighteenth century and involving Queen Anne, portrayed by the icon Olivia Colman in *The Favourite*. When her longstanding friendship with Sarah Churchill, Duchess of Marlborough, came to an end, it was reported that the queen's ex-bestie blackmailed her by threatening to reveal intimate details of their relationship and accused her of keeping 'lesbian favourites' who had influenced her decision-making. To be honest, I'd want to be the queen's favourite too, if it meant she didn't chop off my head. So who can blame them?

A lot of the language we have to describe a person's sexuality and their exploration of it is fairly modern, but we all know that attraction between two people of the same gender has existed throughout history. You may have to look a little harder to find LGBTQIA+ people in times gone by, as many people had to hide their sexuality because of the hugely homophobic laws of the time. Unless we go back really far to Graeco-Roman times where it seems like everyone just openly got off with everyone and lived their best sexy lives, feeding each other grapes while basking in the sun. And even then, it was mostly still male relationships being documented: women were a footnote. Let's face it – as time progressed, our freedom took a big step backwards (it didn't use to be illegal to have abortions – men made it so) as the men of the world continued to cultivate a secret club called the patriarchy, where everyone got persecuted in some way – except them. Funny that. And as if being a woman isn't bad enough, try loving other women on top of that – double the prejudice, double the fun, right?

The earliest known record of a same-gender couple dates back to the twenty-fifth century BC. According to scholars Thomas Dowson and Greg Reeder they were Khnumhotep and Niankhkhnum (great words for Scrabble), which roughly translates to 'joined in life' and 'joined in death', and they were Ancient Egyptian royal servants. They shared the title of

'Overseer of the Manicurists' in the palace of King Nyuserre Ini (not that kind of manicure apparently, but I like to think they were excellent at old timey gels or shellac). They were found buried together in the tomb of King Unas and are listed as 'royal confidants' in their joint tomb. (Who doesn't love a sacred gossip while getting their nails done?)

How do we know they were lovers, you ask? Their bodies were intertwined, and their faces were nose to nose, a tradition that marked the dead as a married couple. Think Romeo and Juliet, but a little more caveman. How *Romeo and Juliet* is still known as the 'greatest ever love story' is beyond me: two fourteen-year-olds (Year 9s!) meet at a party, their parents disapprove, so they throw a strop and pretend to kill themselves for attention. If this is the greatest love story ever told it's in no way rare – Romeos and Juliets exist in every bog-standard secondary school in the UK.

I digress – back to the point – where did it all begin? Where does the term 'lesbian' come from? Well, it literally refers to residents of the Greek island, Lesbos. The island's most famous citizen was a female poet named Sappho, who wrote beautifully romantic poetry about her love for women – so, if Sappho had been residing in Crete, we could have all been cretians! Sappho is thought to have been writing around 600 BC, and while much of her work has since been destroyed due to its mention of lesbianism, she was well respected during her lifetime (she was known as Plato's tenth muse, although it seems a bit rude to be anybody's tenth favourite anything).

Today, we are left with only fragments of Sappho's poetry. Lesbianism, according to Galen, a second-century Greek physician, was caused by an 'ongoing and persistent itch in some women's labia'. The good news? Relief could be had by rubbing your affected labia against that of another woman. How's that for convenient. While you weren't persecuted for being a lesbian, it was still thought of as an illness to be cured. Whereas the men were getting it on and no one was batting an eyelid.

We're unsure when the word lesbian first came into use, because in the Victorian era the word 'sapphists', named after Sappho herself, was used. It's thought to have become more common during this era, when it first appeared in a medical dictionary ('Ah yes, you have a case of lesbianism!' – I hate to think how they tried to cure it). Technically the first lesbian with a capital L on record was Anne Lister – yes, of the story that inspired the hit BBC series *Gentleman Jack*. Back in 1834, Anne was the first woman in England to openly marry another woman – a marriage not recognised under law. Her secret diaries, written between 1806 and 1840, detail her romantic and sexual relationships with women. That said, the word lesbian didn't 'trend', as it were, until as recently as the feminist era of the sixties and seventies, and, girl, since then we've kept it at the top of the hashtag popularity list.

After the Victorian era, some women did live openly, but their sexuality has been ignored or hidden by those who have written about and researched their lives. 'I am reduced to a thing that wants Virginia . . . It is incredible how essential to me you have become,' wrote Vita Sackville-West to the novelist Virginia Woolf in 1926. A successful writer herself, Vita proclaimed her love for Virginia during the 1920s. Although both were married to men, they were openly in love and the two women penned hundreds of poetic letters to each other, and their relationship inspired one of Virginia Woolf's most celebrated works, the 1928 novel *Orlando*. A lot of sexy, cool writers are lesbians . . . just saying. I just need to work on my poetry. Does nothing really rhyme with orange?

Recent examination has suggested that Emily Dickinson was in a romantic relationship with Susan Gilbert, her long-time childhood friend. Susan married Emily's brother (imagine having to sit through that wedding!), but that didn't deter the two from their passionate communication – which was erased when Susan's daughter, Martha Dickinson Bianchi, prepared Emily's letters for publication. As legendary LGBTQIA+ historian Lillian Faderman wrote in *Surpassing the Love of Men*, 'If Emily Dickinson were suspected of lesbianism, the universality and validity of her poetic sentiments might be called into question.' Like Sappho, all over again.

Then there's Mademoiselle Maupin or La Maupin, a famous seventeenth-century sword-slinger and opera singer. Real name Julie d'Aubigny, she was born around 1673 and first started her singing career at the Opéra de Marseille, where she quickly fell for a young woman. The young woman's parents were not at all approving and sent their daughter away to a convent in Avignon. Julie, high on love and passion, followed her lover into nunhood. When one of the other nuns at the convent died, the couple stole the body and placed it in Julie's beloved's cell as a cover. Then they set fire to the convent to cover their tracks and escaped. Because setting fire to buildings is generally illegal, La Maupin was charged with kidnapping, arson and failing to appear before a tribunal. It didn't matter that she didn't show up to court, they still sentenced her to death at the stake! I know we talk about twin flames, but there's love and then *literally* getting set on fire for it. Luckily, she returned to Paris, still alive, and got up to all sorts of mischief, along with duels and becoming the star of the Paris Opéra where she was named La Maupin.

As African-American writer Audre Lorde wrote in *The Master's Tools Will Never Dismantle the Master's House*: 'Those of us who stand outside the circle of this society's definition of acceptable women; those of us who have been forged in the crucibles of difference – those of us who are poor, who are lesbians, who are Black, who are older – know that survival is not an academic skill. It is learning how to take our differences and make them strengths.'

So, like women in general when it comes to history, us lesbians were totally erased unless we were locked in an attic somewhere for allegedly going mad, when actually we were just having a period. How did one explore such longings in times gone past? Conveniently, women were often left alone at home with other women while men went off to . . . shoot . . . do business . . . and do whatever . . . else . . . men do? Watch football? Beats me.

The colour purple

How did women back then know other women had similar longings to them? Well, before American singer-songwriter Olivia Rodrigo made purple cool again by painting her albums lilac, the colour was used to signal a woman's love for other women. Surprising as it may be, the lesbian dress code of the

1920s was not just made up of petticoats and lace-up boots: lesbians also attached sprigs of violets to their lapels like brooches as a sign for other women. This is likely why the colour purple is still associated with lesbian women today, although the shade of choice is now lavender.

I'm trying not to think too hard about how as girls we had two stereotypical options to paint our bedroom walls: pink or purple. Weirdly, I was a pink girl. I clearly missed something there.

When we look at the colour purple throughout history, it makes a strange sort of sense that it's been lovingly adopted by lesbians and the LGBTQIA+ community. For much of history, purple was considered rare when it came to dyes and consequently purple clothing was expensive and often considered a royal colour. People considered purple to be special and something to be celebrated, incredibly fitting for the LGBTQIA+ community. Sappho often wrote of violets, hyacinths and lavender within her poetry: beautiful flowers, adorned in shades of purple that were found, claimed and celebrated even when not typically available to the masses. It's a symbol of lesbian love through history – found and cherished despite the odds.

However, there have been times when purple has also been seen as an undesirable colour and yet even in that, it can sum up our collective experience. In the thirteenth century, violet was designated as the colour used for ceremonies of the dead by Pope Innocent III and became associated with death and was avoided at all costs. Purple represents the 'other', the different or deviant. One of the first lesbians I met and consequently stuck to like glue was so out and proud, she had bright purple hair. I only wished I could have pulled that off.

There are two versions of the lesbian flag, which can you believe was only created in 2018? One has seven stripes and the other has five. Each stripe symbolises an aspect of being queer and wonderful:

Colours on the lesbian flag

Dark orange Gender non-conformity

Orange Independence

Light orange Community

White Unique relationships to womanhood

Pink Serenity and peace

Dusty pink Love and sex

Dark rose Femininity

4
Deconstruction of a lesbian

Dear Diary,

What is a lesbian? I feel like I've been overloaded by societal judgements and expectations of what I should and shouldn't be and I want to shout, 'YOU NEED TO CALM DOWN, YOU'RE BEING TOO LOUD', à la Taylor's banging 'National Anthem'. Does lesbian fit me? I don't think I've grown into it yet. I'm still very much dressing in the kids' section. What can I say, kids' clothes are tax free? I think I'm what my friend Jess would call a Baby Gay. Am I? What is my identity? Where do I fit in this new queer landscape?

Love,
Rosie x

Identity. Now that's a big subject. *Who am I?* I say as I stare in the mirror stabbing myself in the eye with my mascara. It's a life-long journey, I remind myself, with as much zen as I can muster. We are all transcendent, able to change and define ourselves however we feel comfortable.

Thanks to the media there are a whole load of stereotypes and clichés when it comes to being gay. But in general the main thing that makes you gay . . . is liking the same sex. And what makes you bisexual is being attracted to both. Not what clothes you wear, whether you can hit a baseball or build a birdhouse. If these were the criteria I would be laughed out of the interview room. 'Hi, my name's Rosie and I like Taylor Swift, flowery dresses and bows to wear in my hair.' All these stereotypes come from society's idea of gender.

Gender is a social construct that is rooted in the assumed and approved ways people believe men and women should behave. In the simplest terms: the girls get the dolls to play with and the boys get the cars. But when left to their own devices, we know many little boys love a buggy and lots of little girls love running around in the mud with a monster truck.

Society once decided that masculine was naturally supposed to be attracted to feminine. Probably something to do with the Bible and Adam and Eve – and that flipping apple. But 'femininity' and 'masculinity' are meaningless phrases used to perpetuate the idea of heterosexual love, which throughout history was deemed the only way to love.

When someone says the word 'lesbian', what image pops in your head? Growing up for me it was a cropped haircut, baggy T-shirt and looking like I was about to appear in Avril Lavigne's 'Sk8er Boi' music video, mainly due to whatever stereotypical representation the media was peddling feeding into my own subconscious bias – so let's debunk some myths about being a gay woman in the twenty-first century.

'One person must take on the role of a man.'

There's a thought that in any relationship one partner takes the more dominant male role and the other a more female role. This split is again based on gender stereotypes and the way we assign jobs and roles to men and women. I say we take a hammer and smash up this idea. Sure, you might be more confident and the one who likes to take charge – that doesn't make you the man in the relationship. You can figure out how to have balance without conforming to gender stereotypes. It's inherently sexist to suggest that women who are confident or good at DIY are anomalies, and that the ability to put together a bookshelf is something only a man is capable of. Ultimately, you are free to be whoever you want to be in a relationship and this doesn't have anything to do with how you present.

'Lesbians are masculine.'

There are men who are more feminine presenting, there are women who are more masculine. And sure, at times before I really joined the community I worried that there weren't gay women who looked like me. A tiny 5-foot 2-inch ginger girl who likes pinafore dresses. There's lots of ways to present, and none of them determine who you love. Your style and interests don't affect your sexuality, and vice versa.

'Lesbians hate men.'

Just because you don't fancy men – it doesn't mean you can't like them. Hating 50 per cent of the population will get tiring pretty fast. They're around all the time; we can't avoid them. And look, a lot of women have good reason to dislike men.

Many of us have been deeply hurt by their behaviours. When one in four women has been sexually assaulted or raped by a man, it makes sense we might not see them in glowing colours. And while we know it's 'not all men', that statistic is hard to ignore. A recent debate on social media involved women answering whether they would rather be confronted in a forest by a man or a bear, and almost everyone opted for the bear. Because they were less likely to die, and if they were attacked they wouldn't be asked 'What were you wearing?' and 'Why were you walking alone?' Lesbians and men have one major thing in common – our love of females – but it doesn't mean we've got some villainously competitive nature against them.

'Lesbians love sport.'

Absolutely not. Throw a ball. I will not be running. Or catching. I am not a Golden Retriever. My Apple watch has to buzz every few hours to check I'm not in fact dead. Your hobbies have nothing to do with your sexuality or how good you are at DIY or woodwork (another cliché). One time I was building an ottoman bed and managed to trap myself inside it and my neighbours had to come and get me out. Sure, there are women who are amazing at these things . . . but that doesn't make you gay and it's reductive to suggest all lesbians should be good at sport. Do not sign me up for a marathon, thank you.

'Lesbians fancy all women.'

Do your straight friends fancy all men? Heck no. You're allowed to have choice. This is dating, not paying taxes.

'Lesbians and tomboys are the same thing.'

Again. What you wear does not determine your sexuality. LOUDER FOR THE PEOPLE AT THE BACK. You can still shop at Zara.

'People can tell you're a lesbian by looking at you.'

While gaydar is apparently a real thing, it's potentially harmful as it can perpetuate stereotypes of gay women. Although queer people spotting queer people can be quite a lovely thing. My friend Ellen, who is an iconic lesbian, knew I was gay within the first three minutes of meeting me, without me saying a word.

'You can't know you're a lesbian unless you've dated men.'

Some people just know. I have friends who've been out since they were teenagers and have known their whole lives. As someone who's dated both, sure, it made me very sure I didn't want to go near men ever again. But you don't have to experience something to know you don't like it. I've never tried oysters but can guarantee those slimy little poisons are not for me.

'It's a phase, you just haven't met the right guy.'

Oh boy. For a while I wished it was a phase. I wished I could grow out of it. And sure, your sexuality is fluid and maybe you'll want to be with women and maybe with men again, but we're not all out here just dating women because Prince Charming got lost trying to save Fiona from *Shrek* and fell in a creek. The idea that we must all want a man is comical, because if I'm honest I'd rather have a Furby.

Of course, like all things in life, there are some tropes that do ring true for many:

> *'We're lesbians, of course we share each other's wardrobe.'*
>
> *'We're lesbians, of course we're friends with our exes.'*
>
> *'We're lesbians, of course we move in with each other after three months.'*

There is no wrong or right way to do this. There's no rule book. Except this one. Obvs.

So where does sexuality come from?

Is it predetermined? Or is it shaped by our early experiences? A lot of people I know fancied the sexy fox in Disney's *Robin Hood* when they were children, and I'm pretty sure they're not wandering the streets at 1 a.m. lusting after foxes now.

There's a line in the hit Netflix series *Baby Reindeer*, where the main character, Donny, muses on whether, if he hadn't had been abused by a man, he would still find men attractive. It stopped me in my tracks because for me it was the opposite, having been abused by men, I have often wondered whether that meant I found safety and an attraction in women. Sure, we can trace me liking girls back to those very early ballet classes, – did I mention that? – but if men hadn't hurt me, would I have been willing and open to continue to engage in relationships with men? Would I be bisexual rather than gay? Did I buckle down to being gay as a way to make sure men never touched me again? Who knows. But our experience and childhood shape every aspect of our identity, including our sexuality.

The idea that we are born a certain way was posed to counter the conservative belief that people are born straight and homosexuality is a choice – something to be corrected. Until 1979, homosexuality was thought of as a mental illness in the USA. Which is funny because of the amount of mental illness that stems from people not being accepted for who they truly are. If you could just tick a box at the doctor's that read, 'Victim of prejudice because of who I love', wouldn't that be great.

Throughout history, heterosexuality has always been considered the norm. Anything that deviated from this very rigid model was seen as depraved or pointedly referred to as a chosen 'lifestyle'. The work of women who embraced this 'lifestyle' was often cast aside, undervalued or mocked. Anne Lister, Ruth Ellis, Mercedes de Acosta, Jane Addams to name a few. No one would choose to be the outcast. Which is why the LGBTQIA+ community is made up of some of the most welcoming people you could ever wish to meet. We know what it is to be on the sidelines. Lesbians were cast aside in the eye of society; we've been there, fighting from the sidelines, since the beginning.

PART TWO
SEX?

5

What's in a name?

Dear Diary,

I don't even recognise my own name written down, how am I meant to know my identity?

Love,
Rosie x

'So how do you identify?' is a question I still dread, usually posed by a person with a margarita in hand and slightly unfocused eyes. It's all a bit *Mean Girls* and I don't know how to respond. Is it a trick question? Will I live up to whatever answer I give and fit whatever stereotype they hold in their head? I don't know what to say, mainly because it changes on a weekly basis. Not only can I barely recognise my own name when I see it written down (dissociation from myself at its finest), now I have to pick a label. I'm not sure I even have a favourite colour.

Learning about different identities can help you see which one resonates most with your experiences and feelings. Keep in mind that labels are tools for communication but aren't definitive boxes that define your whole being. There is no right or wrong answer to how you choose to identify. And the fluid, evolving, nature of sexuality doesn't always lend itself to definitive declarations.

Labels, labels, labels

Broadly speaking there are five terms for how gay women identify: Lesbian, Gay, Queer, WLW (that's women loving women) sapphic and, of course, there's bisexuality. But there are loads more. It's important to note you can identify with as many, or as few, as you like. It's totally up to you as an individual. It's different for everyone.

But how do you know which one you are? So how do you know what your identity is? I've always assumed that identity must be important given how many hoops I have to jump through to get a new passport, and how often my bank warns me that my identity might be stolen. If anyone wants to be me, please by all means give it a go. A word of warning: I have a broken bedroom window and you will be sharing a bed with three cats – the pleasure is mine.

Sexual identity is not something that you 'pick' in the same way you would choose an outfit or have a preference for a certain food. Instead, it is something you discover over time as you understand your desires, attractions and feelings. Begin by paying attention to your emotions, attractions and fantasies. What kinds of characteristics and qualities are you drawn to? How do you feel in romantic or sexual situations? Your identity can be fluid and change as you grow and experience life, so don't rush to label yourself unless it feels right. Some people identify one way at a certain point in their lives and later discover that their feelings or attractions have evolved. It's completely normal for sexual identity to be fluid, bringing freedom and comfort as you explore who you are. Most importantly, remember that your identity is yours to define, and you have the right to change or evolve it as you learn more about yourself.

Our identities are shaped by many things. As children, our brains learn various ways to keep us safe. Many queer people pick up from a very young age that queerness is neither the norm nor totally accepted, and so we may have suppressed certain feelings and thoughts to keep us from being different and, therefore, safe. The psychoanalyst Erik Erikson believed that adolescence plays a hugely important role in the formation of our identities. He described this stage of life as one of 'identity vs. role confusion' and believed that people who are able to discover and commit to a strong identity emerge with a solid sense of self, while those who struggle may be left wondering who they are as they enter adulthood. As teenagers transition to adulthood, they may begin to feel confused or insecure about themselves and how they fit into society. As they try to find a sense of self, young people may experiment with different roles, activities and behaviours (yes, smoking behind the bike shed does count). According to Erikson, this is important to the process of forming a strong identity and developing a sense of direction in life. Teenagers who are not allowed to explore and test out different identities might be left with what Erikson referred to as 'role confusion'. This is super-valid for people who spent their adolescence hiding who they really are. And just to clarify: when Erikson says committing to a strong identity, he didn't mean the emo phase we all went through.

There are many factors that may contribute to the label you choose. Some girls struggle with accepting 'lesbian' as a term due to connotations of hyper-sexuality. When I was growing up it was also a slur thrown around, a marker of being different or having something wrong with you. Therefore, some people might use 'gay' if that label feels more comfortable.

Others, who are attracted to more than one gender, may feel bisexual is right for them.

Being bisexual was the first port of call for me. For a while I identified as bisexual, using it as a way to explore liking both men and women before slowly realising I wasn't into men. But bisexuality is a standalone, legitimate way to identify – not just a holding pattern, as I had made it.

It's important to mention that bisexual people represent the largest identity group amongst LGBTQIA+ people – both amongst adults and young people – and are often victims of negative stereotyping and prejudice, with people demanding they pick a side or labelling them as overly sexual for liking both men and women. Some people find that if they *don't* come out, people assume they're straight, and that if they *do* come out, they're told 'that doesn't exist', they're 'confused or experimenting' or that 'bisexuality is just a stepping-stone towards being gay or lesbian'. They can be labelled as confused/unsure/undecided or simply erased from existence. What's shocking is that some of this hate comes from within the LGBTQIA+ community, with many bisexuals having bad experiences. When a friend of mine was in an iconic gay bar in London hoping to meet a woman, she was told to 'get out and go home to your boyfriend'. Bi+ is its own valid identity, and so are all of the identities under the bi umbrella.

When it comes to pansexuality, I always think of the wine analogy used in the TV programme *Schitt's Creek*: 'I do drink red wine, but I also drink white wine, and I've been known to sample the occasional rosé, and a couple summers back I tried a Merlot that used to be a chardonnay which got a bit complicated. I like the wine and not the label, does that make sense?'

Pansexuality is an orientation defined by the attraction to individuals regardless of their gender. This means that someone who identifies as pansexual is open to feeling romantic or sexual attraction to people of all gender identities, including men, women, non-binary people, genderqueer people, and anyone else who falls outside traditional gender norms.

What distinguishes pansexuality from other sexual orientations is the emphasis on personality and connection over gender. For pansexual individuals, gender isn't the defining factor in attraction. Instead, it's about the emotional, intellectual, or physical connection they share with someone. This means a pansexual person might find themselves attracted to someone because of their sense of humour, their kindness, or their creativity, not based on whether they fit into a particular gender category.

Just like any other sexual orientation, pansexuality is about the types of connections and relationships a person is drawn to – it doesn't mean that someone is automatically attracted to every person they meet.

When I was exploring my own sexuality, a big question for me was how do you know where on the spectrum I sat? Was I fully committed to women or was I happy to still have men in my (sexual) life? (Can't kick them all out!) Could I be pansexual? Omnisexual? Maybe it won't be until you've been with a woman that you'll know the answer. A lot of people identify as bisexual without having experienced a same-sex relationship, but knowing that they're attracted to the same sex. However you identify, is up to you. For so long, I was so worried about being a fraud. I swear that even if I trained as a neurosurgeon for ten years my brain would convince me I had no idea what I was doing. (If I've learnt anything from my time here on earth it's this: do not believe every thought that comes into your head.)

Identifying as bisexual doesn't mean you have to fit some made-up criteria, such as having a certain percentage of attraction to a particular sex. If you decide on a label there is often a feeling to 'prove it' somehow. But no one should have to prove themselves to be respected for who they are.

A good way I think about it is to imagine myself on the London Underground. When the doors open, some beautiful human is going to step through the space, *X-Factor* style, and I'm going to instantly fall in love with them. I am 98 per cent sure that person is going to be a woman. But I can't guarantee that will be the case for the entirety of my life going forward. When I think about how much I've changed just in my twenties – my thoughts, fears, feelings, expectations – I can't expect myself to be the same at sixty-five. Sure, I'll still have a killer array of Converse and maybe pink hair, but there's a small chance I won't be with a woman. In fact, when a tarot reader recently told me that a very important man was going to walk into my life and change everything . . . I was shaken. She tried to tell me it was a relationship before I mentioned I was gay, and then we settled on him being a business opportunity. Sure, she might be as psychic as my nan, but I can't see the future and I don't know what lies ahead. What I can say is there is no percentage that determines your sexual identity – this isn't GCSE maths where we're on boundary grades. No one is thinking, 'What a shame. If only you'd had one more kiss with a woman, you'd be an A* Lesbian.' There's no one standing at the gates of heaven making sure we are what we say we are, either. How you choose to identify will always be your choice. If you find yourself not wanting to explore with men at all, then that's a good sign you might be gay.

How am I supposed to pick?

Picking a label that fits can feel daunting. Might you be stuck with whichever you choose forever? Like when I said I liked unicorns and spent the next five birthdays and Christmases only getting unicorn-themed presents. Let's be clear: there is no time limit or finish line when it comes to finding out who you are.

I've always struggled with the concept of labelling. For me, it seemed to be something that let other people know where I fit in society. What box I should be put in. But in my head I'm just . . . me? I'm a lot of things. And I don't know if I want to be defined by any of them. And labelling can create a divide between us all. As humans we're ever evolving and ever changing and should be allowed the space to do these things.

If I'm honest, I'm still not sure which label I use to identify. It's like trying on a bunch of jackets and seeing which one fits right. Sure, one might work for spring but it might not cross over come autumn. And that's OK. It's a journey – you don't have to decide and feel like you need to stick to it forever; it's not Peter Pan's shadow waiting to be sewn on to the sole of your foot. I struggled with the term 'lesbian' for a long time. When I was growing up it was a marker of you being different or having something wrong with you. I was made to believe it was a dirty word. Under the umbrella of lesbian there are many 'stereotypes' reflecting underlying distinctions between positive perceptions (lipstick lesbian, career-oriented feminist) and negative perceptions (sexually deviant, angry butch), and I didn't want to be defined by any of them.

Luckily, the term has been celebrated and reclaimed by shows such as *Derry Girls* ('she's a wee lesbian'), and as Georgia on *I Kissed a Girl* once stated, 'L comes first in LGBTQIA+ so why should we be ashamed for saying it?' Maybe it's something I just need to practise saying in front of the mirror three times and then Rihanna will appear from behind it and make out with me.

I spent a lot of time (and still do) trying to figure out which word sums me up best. While sapphic sounds beautifully romantic, a lot of people don't know what that means and I haven't got time to explain Greek history when finding the confidence to speak about my identity. Gay, I quite like, it sounds happy. Delighted. Short, snappy. Queer, though reclaimed by the LGBTQIA+ community, for me still references the time when it meant weird and people were outcast from society. And whereas I could be justifiably described as 'weird' for spending my evenings watching 'What I ate at Disneyland Florida!' TikToks in the bath . . . my sexuality is the least weird thing about me.

I still have to practise getting the word 'gay' out my mouth. Sometimes it comes out too quick, too forceful, like something that doesn't belong to me and I'm trying to make work. I was once in a meeting with a producer who assumed I would meet lots of men at my friend's wedding and would surely get a date. When I went to correct her with 'Oh I'm gay', I said it with so much emphasis an ice cube flipped from my mouth and landed on her plate. I'm trying to convince myself and others at the same time. My friend Helen, a kickass, hilarious woman with excellent style, who's been in a relationship with a woman for years, identifies as 'not straight' which I think is kind of great. Identify as whatever you like, guys! There's no judgement here. Essentially what I'm saying is, don't freak out like I did and think it's the be-all and end-all. You've not just signed up to look after a Tamagotchi.

What I didn't realise at first is that the terms 'baby gay' and 'legendary gay' are often used by the gay community. Readers, I am still very much classified as a baby gay. Exploring this new territory with the wide-eyed wonder of a toddler in soft play . . . just wandering around aimlessly, putting fewer things in my mouth (down, girl). Essentially, in the grand scheme of things, it's all still relatively new and very exciting to me. Then we have people like Miriam Margolyes, Sarah Paulson and my friend, Jess, long in her years of being gay, who all classify as legendary gay. There is nothing these women don't know about being with another woman. I can only assume they were busy being glorious and didn't have time to write this book, so the job has fallen into my lap. I'm wondering if I have to earn badges to allow me to claim that title? Is it like a GAIL's loyalty card where

I get a stamp towards legendary gay every time I date a woman? How many women do I have to date? Is it like hobbies, where if you practise for one thousand hours they say you're an expert? Either way, I'm working my way to that title with the ferocity of a dance mom at Nationals.

6

H is for homophobe

Dear Diary,

Why do people hate me because of who I love?

Love,

Rosie x

I can't deny that when I was coming to terms with liking girls, it made me realise that I had a load of internalised homophobia, and I was frightened of people being homophobic towards me. I'm the kind of person who people expect to move out of the way when they walk towards me on the street. So the idea of being out with a girl and the possibility of someone shouting homophobic slurs at me filled me with terror. I didn't want to be shouted at for being in love. But you can't escape the stories and statistics. There are people not OK with gay people and suddenly, with my newfound freedom, I was having to google where was safe for me to go on holiday. But as a friend said, 'Rosie, in some countries they stone girls for wanting an education, for not wanting arranged marriages. Unless you're planning on actually going to any of these frightening places, you need to get on with being gay.'

Internalised homophobia and oppression happen to us all – no matter our sexual identity – because, as I've already discussed, we have been taught that heterosexuality is the norm and the 'correct way to be'. When we're part of the LGBTQIA+ community, hearing and seeing negative depictions of LGBTQIA+ people can lead us to internalise these messages and make them mean that there's something wrong with us. Witnessing outright homophobia in the media and attacks on our well-being elicits a feeling of being 'othered' by society. If people tell us 'being gay is wrong' we end up with a self-message of 'there is something wrong with me' and carrying round a very large rucksack of shame. Something we have to learn how to put down. Of course, logically I knew there was nothing wrong with being gay at all, but I couldn't make it acceptable for myself.

For a long time I turned the anger I felt about being gay inwards. The dream of my white picket fence and naturally conceived children went up in flames, and there was part of me that was so mad – which was difficult to hold, seeing as women have long been taught not to be angry. Any emotion is preferable to anger. We push it down so it becomes depression, sadness; we let it morph into something else rather than expel it outwards where it belongs. Dr Gabor Maté is a physician who has researched the connection between anger and chronic illnesses, including autoimmune diseases. Maté believes that suppressing anger can lead to the chronic secretion of stress hormones, which can suppress the immune system and lead to autoimmune diseases – and 80 per cent of sufferers are women.

Maté says he can tell when a woman walks into his clinic whether or not they'll fit the bill for an autoimmune issue. He describes these women as Type C personalities: people who suppress negative emotions, especially anger, while maintaining a strong and happy façade. They are people pleasers, extremely cooperative, patient, passive, lacking assertiveness and accepting. As women our anger is constantly made into our own responsibility. We're continually reminded that our emotions risk affecting others – more so than they might affect ourselves.

I know that I run from my own anger; in fact I sprint so fast on a treadmill to avoid it you'd think I was being chased by a sabre-toothed tiger – particularly in cases where the only affected person is myself. I can stand up for other people; it's easier to feel angry on behalf of others who have been treated badly. I can add my anger from my own experiences to their experiences and fight back. I can feel outraged for a friend, I can write strongly worded emails for a colleague. But that's still denying myself my own anger about my own experiences. From the day we're born, girls are taught to care for others far more than we do for ourselves.

We are not taught to defend ourselves. If a man catcalls us in the street, we're urged to 'just take it as a compliment' and move on. If a boy violates us we're told that 'boys will be boys' – we're told if we complain we're ruining their lives. We tend to accept that there's almost no point in calling anyone out because both the perpetrator and society will try to gaslight us into silence by making us feel we're wrong to feel this way. Like we've somehow got the situation totally wrong. While I'm working on my relationship with it I still can't feel anger without feeling that it's my fault and I'm going to get in trouble for it. Even if I say 'I am angry with you' in my most gentle voice, I am still afraid I am too much.

I had to learn to turn the anger about being gay and losing the life I had decided for myself into a whole load of self-compassion. I had to allow all the feelings that came up around being gay to exist, including the anger. If you ignore an emotion, it'll keep showing up until you notice it.

When it came to self-compassion, I learnt there were three elements:

- **Self-kindness instead of self-judgement.** Approaching our experience with non-judgemental curiosity and emotional warmth. A willingness to take care of ourselves.

- **You're not alone in this.** Embracing imperfection and making sense of our experience as a shared human experience. Recognising and understanding others' suffering.

- **Mindfulness instead of over-identification.** Noticing our thoughts and emotions as they are (whether a positive or negative emotion). Not holding on to them nor dismissing them, just letting them exist.

Before I came out I was scared of what people were going to think of me and that was an exhausting weight on my shoulders. It came out as a horribly self-critical voice. I felt I had to overachieve in order to feel accepted. I felt like I had to make up for this part of me. Like 'look at all these perfect, brilliant parts of me, so you don't look and judge my sexuality. Woo look over here, not over there.'

The funny thing is I had tons of male gay friends, but I didn't have many female ones to show me it was not just survivable but an amazing way to live. It was totally OK for everyone else in the world to be gay, but not me. That didn't just extend to my sexuality, but also to my perfectionism, my morality, every which way I lived my life. Everyone else was allowed to do and be whoever they wanted to be with no judgement from me, but I was holding myself to some impossible standard in order to be seen as perfect. Sexuality has no morality, Rosie. Shut up.

I learnt it's OK to have conflicting emotions. BOTH/AND. You can feel pride and happiness and still hold sadness and anger at the ongoing challenges the LGBTQIA+ community faces and your own internal thought pattern.

They're hating you for who you love. They're hating you for your capacity to love. And maybe they're jealous. Like when your mum used to tell you the kids at school were just jealous of your terrible new haircut, they're jealous of your capacity to experience this beautiful, natural feeling that they so desperately want.

In order to undo this way of thinking I had to learn to register and acknowledge my self-judging and critical thoughts when they arose and then correct them. It took a while to develop the awareness of when I was trying to be perfect and to remind myself: it's futile. No one on this planet is perfect, and it's pretty miserable trying to achieve perfection.

The niggle that being gay was wrong sat in my mind for a long time. Luckily, thoughts aren't always true. They're real, you're having them, but that doesn't make them the truth.

I learnt an amazing exercise from Byron Katie, an incredible speaker and author who focuses on self-inquiry, that's helped me with my thoughts. All the suffering that goes on inside our minds is not reality, she says. It's usually the stories we torture ourselves with. Her turnaround method, a system of asking yourself four questions, helped me realise that what I think is simply something I'm choosing and that there are other options.

Here's how the turnaround method helped me with my internalised homophobia.

The turnaround method

The thought It's wrong to be gay.

Question 1 Is it true?

It's not wrong for others but it feels wrong for me.

Question 2 Can you absolutely know it's true?

No. Sexuality is not quantifiable.

Question 3 How do you react when you believe that thought?

I feel sad, alone and filled with shame.

Question 4 Who would you be without that thought?

I would be free to live as I choose. I would be lighter. I would be happy in myself.

Then you turn the thought around It is not wrong to be gay.

The 'turnaround' gives you an opportunity to experience the opposite of what you think you believe. Once you have found a turnaround to your original statement, you are invited to find at least three specific, genuine examples of how the turnaround is true in your life.

- There are lots of amazing women living brilliant lives who are gay.
- I am loved by many people who know that I am gay and aren't prejudiced against me.
- Being gay is literally celebrated with an entire month.

You can use this method with any thought pattern you have, but I found it particularly useful to show how your brain makes up stories about you that aren't true. (Thanks, brain, for being a twelve-year-old girl making up rumours about me!)

Homophobia is ultimately fear

People fear what they don't understand, and I was fearful of people's reactions to and judgements of me when I came out. However, I've been lucky and have experienced very few instances of personal homophobia. When I came out online, I had men in my DMs sending me crass messages about how it was evil, what a disappointment it was – or my personal favourite, 'Can I change your mind?' With your face, sir? Absolutely not. But I have friends who've been the subject of horrific homophobia. We must always remember that we are *not* what happens to us and we are *not* what other people choose to do to us. We cannot allow ourselves to identify with these acts of cruelty. We cannot make them mean something about us. They don't define us (but do tell us a lot about the people who choose to behave in this way) and we deserve the support and love to heal from these things.

Given the amount of homophobia within our society is it any wonder that the LGBTQIA+ community's mental health is suffering? Homophobia isn't always instantly recognisable cruelty: it can take the insidious form of constant micro-aggressions. Having to navigate this kind of ignorant behaviour is something that comes with being part of the LGBTQIA+ community and can take a real toll on your mental health. The world is on fire, we're on the brink of World War III and people are paying £75,000 for a Met Gala ticket. It's no wonder everyone's mental health is already in the bin, without throwing homophobia into the mix. We're on our knees, and in the UK our mental health system is failing us all miserably. With horrifically long waiting lists and doctors uneducated in mental health – we're in a crisis. Put simply, there isn't enough help available for those who need it. A recent national LGBTQIA+ survey by the UK Government revealed that 28 per cent of respondents found it 'not at all easy' to access mental health support. When they did get mental health support, 22 per cent reported a negative experience.

Worryingly, some respondents had been offered harmful treatments such as conversion therapy, most often by faith groups but also by healthcare professionals – despite condemnation of this treatment by major counselling and psychotherapy bodies and the NHS. These challenges also extend to online support. For example, a review of web and mobile phone resources for depression and anxiety suggests that they are largely aimed at heterosexual users and seldom cater for the needs of LGBTQIA+ people. These resources fail to address issues such as coming out and coping with experiences of discrimination or harassment, with few including referrals to mental health services that specifically focus on the queer community.

We need to address the fact that the members of the LGBT-QIA+ community are deeply affected and deserve the help they need. According to a study carried out in 2022 by The Trevor Project, 45 per cent of LGBTQIA+ youth seriously considered committing suicide at least once in the past year. There is a clear need for LGBTQIA+-friendly mental health resources, and finding an LGBTQIA+-friendly therapist is essential for members of the community who are seeking mental health support.

Therapy can change your life

If I were prime minister for the day, the one thing I would promise is that everyone would have access to therapy. I'd be throwing it out like an American game show host. 'You get therapy', 'You get therapy' and 'Everyone gets therapy . . . and a Toyota!' In the US therapy is often covered by health insurance, which is why people have access to a therapist, in the same way they have a doctor. It's normalised. However, in the UK the mental health system is abysmal. On the NHS the wait time to be seen can be years, and then usually you're only offered a set number of sessions. Accessing private therapy is expensive and not accessible for everyone. Few things make me as angry as this: I know that therapy not only changed my life, but saved it. I would hate to think where I would be if I hadn't stomped up the steps to my therapist on that rainy autumn afternoon. At the worst of times there were weeks where she was the only human I was speaking to. Everyone should get to experience the benefit of a safe, therapeutic relationship if they want one.

Although times are a-changin', there can still be a stigma around therapy. I grew up in an environment where we just got on with everything and never spoke about what was going on around us. As children we do our best to survive and interpret the world as our caregivers show us: we don't get a say in it. For me it was to witness everything and stay silent. When I suggested to a friend she go to therapy, she cried, 'But I'm not MAD! I don't need therapy! There's nothing wrong with me!' Firstly, have you seen the world today? None of us are getting out unscathed. But it's such misinformation that there has to be something wrong with you to be in therapy. Therapy can be a mental health workout. You go to the gym or exercise to keep physically fit . . . so why wouldn't you treat your brain the same way?

It's not an entirely bleak landscape; there are therapists who work on sliding scales where you pay what you can, and there are charities that can help with specific issues. When finding help, an important aspect is finding a therapist who is LGBTQIA+ friendly; someone who sees the LGBTQIA+ experience as a lens rather than an issue. Having a therapist who is aware of the nuances of being LGBTQIA+ can make the therapeutic experience more effective. That's not to say you have to see a therapist who is part of the community, just one who's well informed and a friend of the community. Therapy is a space completely for you, and you can use it to explore anything you'd like. It's like having a cheerleader in the corner who's always on your side to help you grow and become the person you've always wanted to be.

Going to therapy is a quiet act of self-love. You may gawp at that sentence. But turning up to therapy is showing up for yourself and knowing you deserve help and support. We're all made up of many different parts, and while there might be a part of you that thinks self-love is the last thing on your agenda, there is a tiny part of you that is there cheering you on. If you're trying to love yourself then deep down you already do, and that's a good place to start.

Because ultimately it is up to us. A large part of therapy is giving you back the autonomy in your life, now that you're an adult. The only person who's going to save you, is you. So many of us dream of someone coming along and solving everything, being looked after, being treated well. Life would just be better if that person turned up. But it's a set-up to fail. We need to have our own backs.

When you've been walking a path for so long it can seem impossible, or even dangerous, to veer off it. If you're like me, you try to wait for exactly the right conditions to do something. I thought I needed to be perfectly healed in order to date. Healing isn't linear and it takes time – it doesn't mean you have to miss out on your life in the process.

You might think, but what am I going to talk to my therapist about? Nothing *that* bad has happened in my life (plot twist – most people think that). Maybe you don't have anxiety or depression or what you think people are going to therapy for. There's no end of things you can take to therapy. In general therapy looks at re-parenting you, undoing all the subconscious messages, beliefs and thoughts you've taken in from your environment and, with the help of neuroplasticity, creating new neural pathways so you literally think differently. You can work through past traumas that may be playing a subconscious role in how you show up in day-to-day life, look at behaviours that aren't serving you any more, learn how to process and feel your emotions, explore your identity, build resilience in the face of adversity, all the while being validated and accepted.

7

I can't think straight

Dear Diary,

I want to be good. I want to be thin. I want to be perfect. Maybe I should start recording my weight, my cigarettes and my sexual conquests à la Bridget Jones. I've somehow assigned morality to everything and I'm struggling to cope under the weight of wanting to be 'good' all the time. If I start assigning goodness to my identity, then I know I'll end up in trouble. I want to be a good person, who makes enough money to look after my cats, who has a thriving social life, while being politically informed, fighting the patriarchy, doing weekly activities and in a banging relationship, and ignore the impending doom that sits in my stomach every time I read the news. Simple, right? This spiral I'm in now feels never-ending and I'm coping in ways that aren't healthy.

Love,
Rosie x

Women and our bodies: a duo more iconic than Thelma and Louise. Throughout history we have been told how our bodies should look, work, and heal . . . by men. It baffles me that there is a gender health gap, with women regularly receiving poorer healthcare than men. Women's healthcare has never been a priority in science which is why I can only assume we're still using a speculum designed in 1845. We have AI and regularly update the software on our phones . . . but no one has decided to update that?

My body and I have had a tumultuous relationship at best that has affected many parts of my life. When you're at war with the vessel that's driving your life, it gets complicated. Take a moment: has your relationship with your body affected your ability to be present in relationships both emotionally and physically? I had to learn how to reconnect with my body and in doing so my sexuality. This section handles subject matters that may be tricky, so please flick forward if you find it upsetting.

Fun fact: food and sex are related. Food and sex are physically connected in the limbic system of the brain, by the hypothalamus which generally controls emotional activity. They walk a similar emotional line and bring out similar types of reactions. To most people they both elicit dopamine. But even before I learnt that little scientific nugget, I had thought that the two must be linked.

I stopped eating after I was sexually assaulted. They say eating disorders can be ticking time bombs lying dormant until something detonates. I didn't even notice at first, or maybe I did and I can't remember. After my assault, which is touched on a little more later in the book, I just wanted to be invisible and take up as little room as possible. I wanted to be cut off from my body that was hurting, physically and emotionally. In order to be safe, I needed to disappear. I needed to be numb.

We frequently ignore the signals our bodies give us. How many times have you been tired but just carried on? When have you needed to pee but resisted going straight to the toilet because you wanted to finish your task first? Have you ever felt your stomach tighten when asked to do something that makes you feel uncomfortable? Our bodies are always talking to us, as they know exactly what they need. The message is clear. It's just that we often cut ourselves off from them.

In my case there was no message to eat, no message to go to bed, no thirst. Eventually a coffee during the day and a meal in the evening became normal for me and I no longer felt hunger. My body stopped giving me signals. I didn't have the energy to flirt, let alone date (I was still funny, though: it took a lot of trauma to come up with this sense of humour). I couldn't even feel turned on by a bar of chocolate . . . how was I going to feel turned on by someone else? Relationships went on the back burner while a newfound eating disorder took centre stage.

Being gay, having an eating disorder and being a survivor of sexual abuse was quite a tightrope to walk and I'd labelled myself 'a breakdown waiting to happen'. After I was sexually assaulted and starving, I stumbled into situations that turned abusive, and the cycle of abuse and not eating continued. As Lucia Osborne-Crowley writes in her incredible book, *My Body Keeps Your Secrets*: prior victimisation is the biggest indicator of future abuse. Do not blame yourself for cycles. It wasn't until escaping that I could fully face my sexuality, my eating disorder and the abuse I'd been subjected to at different points in my life, and end that cycle. Luckily, for me and anyone around me, the layers peeled back one at a time. Thanks to my initial denial of each situation and sheer pure luck on timing, I didn't have to face everything all at once.

The one thing all three had in common? I hated myself for them. And the other thing? None of them was my fault. I had so much shame around what men had done to me, tied up with the confusion of being gay (and would I still be gay if I'd never had the experiences I'd had? Will there ever be an answer to that?), that my coping mechanism didn't exist. And the best way to not exist was to take everything out on my body and try to make it as small as possible.

Until one day my friend, trying to lose weight for her wedding, said to me, 'I've been on a diet, not eating as much and I feel like shit. I realised that must be how you feel all the time.' I didn't know how I felt all the time. I couldn't remember a time when I felt anything. When I didn't feel like this. Tired but pepped up by sugar-laced coffee and a couple of biscuits.

I needed an appetite not just for food. For sex, too.

As I slowly learnt to eat again, I adopted the monotonous regime of three-hour fuelling, a lot of milk-based drinks and measuring pasta into cups. This was all with the help of a dietician and an incredible therapist.

Eating disorder clinics are wild places. I remember being greeted by a teenage girl who marched out of her appointment, slammed the door of the consulting room and shouted, 'Thank you for your advice but I'm not doing ANY OF THAT', before pounding her way down the four flights of stairs. Making girls with eating disorders walk up many flights of stairs seems counter-productive – we love a calorie-burning workout. My eating disorder voice was screaming: yass girl, get those steps in. I was not the only one doing sly lunges in the waiting room.

During an appointment, the dietician asked me if I was sexually active. (I wasn't sure what that had to do with my meal plan.)

'Um . . . not really. I have no appetite for anything.'

'You have to feed yourself. Not just with food. With life. You can't just sit around pretending not to be alive.'

To me my sexuality was dangerous. I couldn't have an appetite. And I certainly couldn't have a sexual appetite.

The problem was that my repressed sexuality was playing a role in my eating disorder. Understanding eating disorders amongst LGBTQIA+ people is about recognising the whole array of factors that might be implicated in the most human of experiences: being in a body. I was trying to control unwanted impulses, both sexual and food-related. Things I deemed unacceptable. I wanted my body to be straight. And by performing as a straight woman, I had to be acceptable as one – and for so long what have we expected of a woman's body? That's right. A thin one.

It makes sense then that Beat, one of the leading eating disorder charities, reports that lesbian, gay, bisexual, transgender people and others in the community are disproportionately affected by eating disorders, and it's generally thought if you're part of the LGBTQIA+ community you're twice as likely to suffer a mental health problem. (Just a disclaimer: being LGBTQIA+ neither causes mental health problems nor means you may have them: it's just that we have a lot of things to handle.)

The reasons why members of the LGBTQIA+ community are more likely to have mental health issues is complicated. But much of it is to do with homophobia, discrimination, rejection and the feeling of isolation. For a long time I felt different. And if you're othered, when you feel like you don't fit in and have no one to talk to, you're going to feel rubbish. Looking after your mental health is important for everyone, but especially so when your sexuality can be weaponised. When there are people who'd rather have you dead than be in love . . . It's not exactly the nicest thing to walk round with in the back of your mind.

There are many ways in which we can take care of our mental health, including the following.

Unplugging

Every day the news and our social media is filled with endless stories of human rights violations, anti-LGBTQIA+ legislations, discriminatory acts, hate crimes and violence against the LGBTQIA+ community. While we can't pretend these things aren't happening, the constant processing of negative news can play havoc with your mental health. We weren't designed to be exposed to a constant stream of information that can elicit feelings of hopelessness, anger, sadness and fear, and the long-term impact of such does damage to our mental health. Try and connect to your body and see how your social media and news consumption is affecting you. Sometimes it's good to take a break and unplug, or set yourself a time limit for how long you're allowed to scroll every day. (Let's not talk about my seven-hour phone consumption I get reminded of every Monday . . .) Protect yourself against accounts and feeds that post distressing information and curate a feed which is for you and is balanced.

Connection

We don't have to go through life alone, and often there's someone out there who feels just like you. Whether you're dealing with unaccepting family members, don't know anyone else in the LGBTQIA+ community, or are looking to connect with others about a particular social issue, there are plenty of LGBTQIA+ groups and communities, both in person and online, that will accept you as you are and can relate to what you're going through. Having people you can talk to and feel seen by is hugely important to your mental well-being.

Prioritise your well-being

The mind/body connection is real! Exercising a little every day does make us feel better, even if it's just going for a short walk. Walking helps boost your mood because it increases blood flow and blood circulation to the brain and body. It has a positive influence on your hypothalamic-pituitary-adrenal (HPA) axis, which is your central nervous response system. This is good because the HPA axis is responsible for your stress response. When you exercise by walking, you calm your nerves, which can make you feel less stressed.

But on the flip side, embracing who you really are can have a wonderful effect on how you feel. Having the freedom of self-expression and self-acceptance can increase your confidence and sense of belonging and – as I found after coming out – hugely improve your mental health and quality of life.

Like sexuality, mental health is a lifelong journey and navigating it can go in peaks and troughs. Nothing lasts forever, the good or the bad. The more I try to live in the present moment, the more I try to stay connected with friends and other members of the LGBTQIA+ community, the easier it gets. In the words of the Academy-award-worthy movie *High School Musical*, 'We're all in this together.' The ordeal of living is a collaborative one. So come share my cake with me.

We'll learn how to accept ourselves, together.

8

13 Going on 30

Dear Diary,

When did everyone get so far ahead? I've looked around and they've Looney Tunes sprinted off in front of me with just tumbleweed left behind. They're graduating college and I'm still in nursery. I'm going to write a book called All My Friends Are Getting Married and I'm Learning How to Eat. The weekend two of my friends got hitched, I got put on a meal plan and while I was measuring out spoonfuls of peanut butter, they were making vows promising no more parking tickets and to pick the wet towels up off the bathroom floor.

I know on the outside it looks like I'm doing OK, but I can't help but notice how painfully single I am. Good job, good apartment, good friends, I just don't have anyone to enjoy life with. What's the point of it all, if you're climbing the mountain alone? I miss the companionship of just knowing that there's someone there. There's only so many times I can text my best friend all my inner thoughts. Am I not meant to have this figured out by now? Isn't that what your twenties are for?

Today I was sitting in a business meeting with my friends Laura and Ruby, in a chic boardroom in Soho, and I couldn't even think straight because all I could think about was how I'm not like them. Laura's had her second baby, Ruby's just got married, they're both dressed in classy outfits that look like they've been lifted right off the mannequins from designer shop windows that I can't afford and I'm wearing a Lizzie McGuire T-shirt. Don't get me wrong, Lizzie is iconic, but I felt so out of place. Why do I feel so goddamn behind them?

I feel so desperately lonely. There's that quote by the American writer Charles Bukowski, which goes something like, 'When there's no one to wake up next to and no one to come home to what do you call it? Freedom or loneliness?' How am I ever going to find my person if only 6 per cent of the population is gay? I can't do the maths in terms of seven billion (i.e. the global population), but it feels like a very small number. I suddenly feel the clock ticking in a way I haven't before. I'm going to have to freeze my eggs (and I don't mean the ones from Sainsbury's). Because Ruby and Laura are both straight it just seems so much easier for them. They've haven't had to have this confusing, tumultuous rebirth and try to find their identity in their twenties. How do I get rid of this feeling that I'm failing in life because I don't have someone to share it with? I mean they taught us that Bridget Jones with her sexy London flat, amazing journalist job and two gorgeous men fighting over her was failing – is it any wonder I feel bad about myself? I want to be the gay Bridget Jones please. I want two hot women fighting in a restaurant over me and declaring their undying love in the snow. Thanks.

Love,
Rosie x

Ever had that panic? For me it usually sets in around 11 p.m. when I catch a glimpse of myself in bed with my Disney pyjamas, spot cream all over my face and even my cat doesn't want to hug me. When I wake up in the morning it's usually passed and I remember, rationally, that it's OK not to have it all figured out. As Phoebe says in *Friends*, when asked if she has a life plan, 'I don't even have a pla!!' Life isn't like it was for our parents and grandparents. Nowadays, thirty doesn't mean you're automatically a spinster destined for the attic with no hope of finding love. We've reclaimed our autonomy, our girlhood. Girlhood is no longer a temporary phase of childhood reserved for summer holidays and Year 8 cliques, but a style of living for anyone who wants to relish in excitement, live authentically and stand up for what they believe in. It's different for everyone, but for me included making A LOT of friendship bracelets last summer. In the past we've abandoned girlhood almost immediately after we leave school because we start to develop a fear of falling behind our friends.

But 'behind' isn't a feeling. Behind the feeling of behind (still with me?) is a whole load of shame for what we think we should be doing. For the first eighteen years of our lives we're pretty much all on the same trajectory. We're hitting milestones generally around the same time as our classmates and can see pretty easily where we fall amongst our peers.

Cut to: 'YOU'RE ON YOUR OWN, KID.' Off you go, hope you survive! Once we leave school, we don't have uniform indicators of measuring progress any more so we end up comparing ourselves to our friends and obsess over how we fall short – how 'behind' we are. This starts as a teenager when everything feels an absolute mess and you're almost in constant competition with your friends over who's the best liked, who's dated the most, who's doing the best in exams, etc. While the things we're comparing may change over time, the essence of the process is the same. I think that perhaps what changes is how much pressure you put on yourself. The younger you are, the more anything seems possible, but as time passes and you see other people who are seemingly 'more successful' you start to feel like you've fallen behind. This is entirely based on external things we can see, like promotions, marriages, kids, houses or – God forbid – how many followers your dog's Instagram account has.

One of the reasons women feel like they're falling behind is a concept entrenched in toxic monogamy called the 'relationship escalator'. The relationship escalator says that all 'legitimate' relationships follow the same trajectory: dating → buying a property → getting married → having children → till death do us part, etc., etc. Reader, we do not have to follow that route. I'd like some music festivals, gazing at the stars, falling off Lime bikes, relocating to New Orleans and some big arguments where I can listen to Adele thrown in, please. The reason I was unhappy before wasn't because I was 'behind' . . . it was because I didn't know how to measure my life according to the things that actually matter to me. How many iced coffee chats did I have that week? Did I make people laugh? Did I stand up for myself in a way I hadn't before? How many bracelets did I sit and make when I was definitely supposed to be doing work, but it's OK because they look fire? You're not allowed to compare your life to someone else's social media highlight reel because you have no idea how that person measures up to your personal criteria for success. It's all relative to what's important to you and doing it in your own time.

Something I think about a lot is . . . what is time? Who invented time? David Tennant? Not to get all *Doctor Who*, but we've sort of made it up, what with putting clocks backwards and forwards and New Zealand being a day ahead of us. It's basically just a concept to make sure we're all awake during sunlight hours and in bed when the predatory foxes of north London are about. Who makes the rules? Go get those pancakes at 3 a.m. There is no right way to live life, but thinking there is a right way is the wrong way. And if there's one thing all the gays know is that we are on our own timeline. Please enter: second adolescence, with all the intense feelings, hormones and excitement that it brings. And I'm just as lost as the first time around. Unfortunately, I can't guarantee this involves less bleeding through skirts and crying in the bathrooms – but at least now we're old enough that we don't have to ask to go to the toilet.

Second adolescence

The result of going through adolescence in a society that still has many prejudices against the LGBTQIA+ community means that many of us didn't feel safe to explore this period of change as our true selves. Many of us hid our identities (or maybe we couldn't yet make sense of how we felt) and consequently many things were pushed down, creating a false self (that's safe but divorced from our true self). And that's how we navigated our teenage years. So, psychologically, our development was interrupted in a way that it wasn't for our straight-presenting peers, resulting in two main impacts: missing out on integral psychological and social developmental experiences (such as first relationships and exploring your wants and needs) and experiencing the trauma caused by an anti-queer society. Of course, there will be people reading this who had supportive, gleeful adolescences, but for the majority of us there were barriers that got in the way of us growing into our healthy, true selves.

So once we start exploring and living authentically, many of us feel undeveloped, confused and behind our straight friends. Especially when you have to start at square one and explore your sexuality all over again. (Pretending to kiss the back of oranges with your friends didn't cut it for you either, huh?) It feels like being thirteen again because psychologically we are. That thirteen-year-old girl, who never got a chance to fully explore her identity, still lives inside you and has finally been given the space to be free. It's sort of like giving a teenage girl your credit card and telling them to go wild.

In order to grow we need to address the experiences our teenage selves missed. The fun part is actually giving yourself those missed experiences. Going on dates, having first kisses, exploring sexually, dressing how you want and living authentically. And if you want to kiss a girl around the back of the cinema after watching a Marvel film to make it really authentic – go for it (at least this time your mum won't be waiting to pick you up)! The harder part is confronting what it means to have missed those experiences the first time round. This can bring up a lot of feelings of sadness and even grief for what you've lost, but those feelings don't last forever. Reframing our experience of 'feeling behind' as going through a second adolescence instead can offer us much-needed validation. It reminds us that although we didn't have the same experience as our peers growing up, that's OK and we are on our own path. It also makes exploring your sexuality a bit easier knowing you're doing experiencing for the first time, exactly like a teenager. Don't hold yourself to 'adult' standards. Allowing the need for a second adolescence gives us empathy for ourselves and our past behaviours.

Sarah speaks of the challenges of a publicly visible timeline of being a twenty-eight-year-old in a suit and heels, but feeling as if she was sixteen again upon coming out – with all the intense, raging emotions, desire to shout 'fuck it' into the wind and do whatever she wanted while keeping it all a secret from her friends and family. Surprisingly, she found the shame and feeling of unworthiness from her teenage years suddenly cropping up again and couldn't understand why, when she was living authentically. Her heterosexual friends were settling down, and she was exploring hook-ups and sexual expression. Once she'd had some (what she considered) wild experiences where she accepted that she was searching for the love she had desired and been denied growing up, she felt herself settle. She realised she was caring for a very young teenager who wanted to be heard, validated and loved. She learnt to move through her old ways and patterns and approach her relationships from a healthy adult standpoint of expressing her needs, boundaries and emotions.

The caveat to second adolescence: it doesn't give you the right to be a dick. We are in our adult bodies and we won't be treating others badly, throwing tantrums or being rude because we're 'now teenagers again'. However, all the fun parts . . . feel free to indulge. And there were some very fun parts to being thirteen.

I essentially approached it like the plot of *13 Going on 30*. Like a kid having fun I allowed myself all the things my teenage self didn't get to have: the clothes, the make-up, the self-love, the grace to try new things and make mistakes, just because I could. I realised that no one was really watching me. Everyone is their own main character in their story and I was just a side plot to them; sure, the focus might shift to me for a second, but in the movie of their life it very quickly reverted to them when I exited the scene. I found freedom without judgement. I allowed myself to have experiences I desperately wanted but didn't get to have. I'm still exploring my way through it with all the excitement and gall of a teenager but with a bit more self-awareness and compassion this time around, and it's allowing me to be a much more responsible adult because of it. Because I've ticked off the appropriate developmental stages that allow me to navigate adulthood successfully.

That doesn't mean it's all plain sailing. So when things get overwhelming, when the little comparison demon comes and sits on my shoulder, I remind myself:

- It's OK to take detours.
- It's OK to be a work in progress.
- It's OK to bloom at your own pace.
- It's OK not to have it all figured out right now.
- It's OK to take your time.

9

It's time to choose you

Dear Diary,

There's something heavy constricting my chest; an old, cast-iron corset I can't escape from. But if this metal bondage fell away, it feels like a scream would break loose, a scream that might never stop. The days have felt muted and grey for a while now. I stumble, fuzzy-headed, through life, half the time side-swiped by memories of my trauma, and the other half I'm too tired to think. I find comfort in reruns of old Disney shows I watch at 2 a.m. when I'm too tired but can't sleep. I have full conversations with people, smile plastered across my face, while my mind is somewhere else entirely.

Today, I'm sitting curled up on my therapist's sofa, clutching my favourite pillow of hers that I've smeared with so much mascara and foundation over the years that there's just a print of my face on it. She tells me there's a very little girl inside me who needs to be seen, who needs to be heard and needs to be loved. I'm frustrated that I can't see her. Not yet, she says, but you will. Through the tears I tell her I feel like I have two options. My voice sounds so young as the words slip through my lips, as if I've been transported back to the kitchen table as a toddler. Either the bad experiences win or I do. There's a pause that hangs in the air, I'm too scared to look up

at her. Her next sentence reaches into my soul and to the little girl
sitting silently alone in her bedroom.

    Please choose you, she whispers. Choose her.

    So slowly, I learn how to.

Love,
Rosie x

If we're accepting our second adolescence we're actually doing what is known as inner child work. Yes, it's the same thing as when Kendall Jenner put a baby photo of herself as her lock screen and everyone else started doing it. But do you know what? That's a great way to start. It's essentially reconnecting with our younger selves who didn't get the nurture and care they needed. Something us LGBTQIA+ girlies need desperately. When I think of younger me, I see a tiny little girl in a blue-patterned school dress with a lopsided fringe (yes . . . the scissors were too inviting – fringes were on trend even when I was four), who is desperate for any kind of attention and will keep playing up until I give it to her.

Taking care of your inner child

Have you ever heard a little voice inside you? One that reminds you of your younger self? One that gets excited at the prospect of Christmas or when you spot your favourite dessert on a menu? Or one that gets awfully upset when it feels ignored? No matter how old we are, we carry our younger selves with us every day. I've always liked the expression 'I am all the ages I have ever been – all at once.' So while you may be thirty-two, you're also twenty-one, ten and five. Just like growth rings inside a tree. Perhaps our hurt six-year-old self shows up when our best friend doesn't text back, and our angsty, misunderstood fifteen-year-old self appears in an argument with a colleague.

Our brains associate experiences and tie together memories and feelings that relate to each other. When your brain recognises a similar situation to one stored as a memory, it brings up those same feelings that are attached to the memory. The stronger your memory – whether it is associated with happiness, fear or curiosity – the stronger the emotional response will be if you find yourself in a similar situation. This is why we often react to experiences in similar ways time and time again: our brains love a pattern. It's near impossible for our brains to create a whole new emotion for each and every experience, so we draw on ones from the past.

Imagine a situation where you feel ashamed because you forgot to complete a piece of work. You may have a disproportionate reaction, perhaps crying hysterically. It's likely your inner child is activated and it remembers being shamed by a parent. When we are treated unfairly as an adult, we are transported back to that feeling of hopelessness and powerlessness we had in childhood.

You may notice that you're experiencing fear, perfectionism, anxiety or are avoiding certain people, places or experiences. These are all ways that your inner child is attempting to feel safe. When your inner child is running the show, they'll choose behaviours, choices and thoughts based on beliefs or memories from the past, based on what they thought they would need to feel safe. Our past always informs our present.

Caring for this younger version of ourselves is what inner child work is all about. This is so often the adaptive child; the child who learnt to survive and navigate the world the best they could is driving the car of our life. We need to take their hands off the wheel, as our younger behaviours may not serve us any more and may instead become destructive. Remember, our inner child is not yet old enough for a driver's licence, and no one needs an angry five-year-old driving a car!

We don't need to abandon ourselves any more. We need to be able to hold every part of ourselves. There are no parents to impress, no need to hide who we are, we can be free to live as we are. We abandon ourselves in many ways, without even realising it.

- Saying yes when you really want to say no.
- Saying yes too quickly without thinking something through.
- Saying sorry when they're the ones who should be apologising.
- Accepting breadcrumbs from people (i.e. the bare minimum).
- Never asking for help.
- Not feeding yourself.
- Not going to the bathroom when you need to.
- Not keeping promises you made to yourself.
- Chasing people who ignore you.
- Not allowing time for sleep.

- Over-explaining everything.
- Going back to situations that do not serve you.
- Not allowing time for rest and relaxation.
- Not speaking up when someone disrespects you.
- Lying to yourself and to others.
- Not taking care of yourself.

By healing our inner child we begin to create the safety and security we always needed. We then can feel safe to reach for connection, to date, to enter a relationship from a safe and solid foundation. When our inner child feels safe, seen and heard the impact on our life is huge – it means we can navigate through the world from our adult self.

So how do we go back and help our inner child? Do we go full *Freaky Friday* and switch places? Not exactly, but we do need to go back into our past and visit them (a bit like *A Christmas Carol*, but cuter).

Because if you're struggling with being gay, it's not something that just rocked up one morning. It's rooted somewhere in your childhood experience.

It's easy to believe that once you find a perfect partner, everything will finally be alright and you'll never have any issues ever again, as if a fairy godmother has waved a magic wand and your life will now be perfect . . . and no bad feelings will ever arise again . . . when actually there's two of you to navigate the chaos of life and double the 'fun'.

A partner is usually a Band-Aid solution. Other people only comfort your inner child as long as they act according to your expectations. The moment they do something that you don't expect, old wounds are brought to the surface and you're in pain again. Maybe they ignore your messages or don't invite you out with their friends, and suddenly you're eight years old and alone in the playground again.

That's why inner child work is so powerful. It allows you to become your own parent and you learn to give yourself as much loving attention as you require to heal. So how do we do it?

1   Firstly we need to acknowledge our inner child. As long as little you gets ignored, we can't begin to help or heal her. To do this I imagine sitting with my younger self. When at first I couldn't imagine her, I imagined a child I had in my life, such as a friend's child or a young cousin.

2   Then we can start communicating with her. Finding a way to hear what your inner child has to tell you is key to accessing the source of any pain, sadness or trauma. Can you listen to what she has to say? How does she feel? What would she like you to do now?

3   Finally, as an adult, you can step into the role of a nurturing parent. Can you tell her you love her no matter what and won't leave her? Your adult self can give your child self exactly what she needs. For me that often meant doing all the things I didn't get to do much of as a child. Activities like bowling and ice skating and spending far too much money in Hamleys buying toys for myself. It's self-love in its purest form.

There are lots of ways we can take care of our inner child.

- Buying things you couldn't afford or weren't allowed as a child.
- Standing up to family members or people of authority.
- Creating a safe space to live in.
- Tuning in and being honest about how you feel about situations and making decisions that are right for you.
- Allowing yourself all your emotions.
- Getting back into films, hobbies and interests you used to love when you were younger.
- Allowing yourself time to play or to be without the pressure of 'adulting'.

We need to acknowledge that this work takes time. For a long time I couldn't do it, I couldn't see my inner child. I didn't want to acknowledge my past and how it was affecting my current life. And then when I did start communicating with her, I got very angry and chopped up loads of photos of me when I was little – which was not the point of the exercise. I had to learn compassion for little me and not to turn away from myself. But once I learnt how to accept her, I could learn how to accept adult me.

The fact that I'm gay is just another facet of who I am. I can accept other aspects of myself – I'm creative, excitable, have two legs and blue eyes – so why can it be so hard to accept the fact that I'm gay?

I was introduced to a Buddhist concept called radical acceptance in 2023, which is your ability to accept situations outside your control without judging the situation, which then reduces the suffering caused by them. Practically speaking, it means acknowledging a lot of difficult situations and emotions. Fully accepting things as they are instead of pushing them aside or wishing for a situation to be different can help us live more freely. Instead of getting caught up in an emotional reaction to what is your reality and prolonging your suffering, radical acceptance allows you to make peace with the situation and move on. Your friend cancels on you last minute: you can be disappointed and annoyed, but after witnessing those emotions you can move on and choose not to let that ruin your evening. I am gay: I can witness the uncomfortable emotions that arise around that statement due to society's expectations and prejudices, but not let them ruin my mental health.

It's all about emboldening yourself to not give your power away. Now I live as openly as I do, there's a lightness to my body that wasn't there before. Holding in secrets feels heavy. Anticipating people's judgements is exhausting and it's really hard to navigate the world hiding your true self.

Choosing yourself is one of the most powerful acts of self-care, growth and empowerment. It's about prioritising your own well-being, values and goals, even in the face of external pressures or societal expectations. When you choose yourself, you are affirming your right to live authentically and to make decisions that align with your true desires and aspirations. But choosing *you* can come with anxiety.

Anxiety – a bit like your inner child – is like a toddler. A toddler who has needs, who wants to be seen, heard, loved, validated. Often when a toddler has a need they'll throw a tantrum.

Anxiety is similar. It can go wild in our bodies (racing heart rate, sweating) and in our brains (spiralling, catastrophising) until we meet the need. Sometimes the tantrum needs to be ignored; at other times it needs love, acceptance and validation. Anxiety is the same: it might need to be witnessed, comforted and accepted in a compassionate way.

Let everything happen to you, the beauty and the terror. It's going to happen anyway, and the more you fight it, the worse it's going to be. A bit like that plant in *Harry Potter* when Hermione tells the boys not to panic, and then Ron gets stuck and she despairs, 'He's panicking, isn't he?' You have to keep going and move through the feelings you're going to have around this section of your life, and there are going to be a lot of them. I like to think of feelings as waves. I'm the ocean. The waves come in, they retreat. Nothing lasts forever – except perhaps the regret that you've waited so long to choose to live your life for you.

10

Throwing out your closet

Dear Diary,

I'm going to wet myself or be sick, or maybe both at the same time. My hands are shaking as I wait for the ancient Boots printer to drop photos of my history into the grimy plastic tray. I've decided to pay an extortionate amount of money to print out photos of my life and take them to therapy to try and help me talk about things. The world must have decided today is the day, because the Boots printer is actually working, which quite frankly is a miracle of its own. I slip the photos into the little, free paper jacket and tuck them in my pocket next to my marathon running heartbeat.

My therapist and I sit on the rug on her floor, and I begin to lay out the photos. I'm wearing my retro Winnie the Pooh jumper, a signal which we've both learnt means 'important, tough session ahead' or 'Babe, I'm having a breakdown'. There's something child-like and comforting about having a giant yellow bear on your chest. We talk through the photos of my friends, me at different stages of my life, photos that circle around events of my trauma that my therapist connects with the ease and agility of a whippet. The patterns of my childhood laid out before me. Then we get to the final one. I flip it over as if I'm playing Snap and quickly turn my head away to stare out the window. I can't look at her.

As she gently asks, 'And who's this?' she's staring at a photo of twenty-four-year-old me, head resting against a beautiful girl, us both pulling stupid faces. We're sitting on a balcony in Gran Canaria. The sun's setting and my hair's wet and it's a captured moment of intimacy that is hard to put into words. A time where everything just felt . . . right? That feeling when you're on holiday between being in the sun all day and getting dressed up to go out for dinner? Knowing there's no stress or alarm clocks or anything but each other?

I take a deep breath, thinking it's now or never . . . but would it be so bad if I just flung myself out the window into the car park?

'I think . . . that's the only person I've ever truly been in love with. I think I might be gay.'

I'm still staring out the window. The car park is suddenly fascinating. I read the make of cars as if that's something I'm interested in. Maybe I'll get a Fiat 500. Maybe I'll die in a car crash. My brain is playing out quick scenarios to distract me from what's just come out of my mouth. I'm waiting to be told off. I'm waiting to be told 'Are you sure? Really?' I'm waiting to be asked to leave.

Instead, I'm met with a very gentle 'Tell me about her.'

I turn back to face my therapist and slowly look up at her. I'm met with the biggest, warmest smile I have ever seen. We talk about her and I explain how frightened I've been to have this conversation.

It's the beginning of us figuring out my sexuality. Of us talking and giving me the confidence to reveal this part of myself to the world. It's a minutely slow process. Millimetre by millimetre. As she says: you can only go as fast as the slowest part of you feels safe to.

If she hadn't responded with such kindness, I wouldn't be writing this now.

Love,
Rosie x

In our white, straight, patriarchal society, the toughest thing about being a lesbian is that you have to be both gay *and* a woman/non-binary. Two attributes that in our white, straight, patriarchal society place us firmly at the bottom of the food chain.

Coming out usually means realising you are LGBTQIA+ (coming out to yourself is a really important first step), and/or telling people you are LGBTQIA+. Coming out can be a brilliant, positive experience, but it may affect your relationships with the people around you if they don't understand or are not supportive. Some people have good experiences of coming out, some have bad experiences, some have an experience that is somewhere in between. It's a sliding scale, but what's important is doing what feels right for you. And maybe you don't know what that is yet. Sexual exploration is a journey, and you don't have to have the answers all at once.

For me, as I mentioned earlier, societal internalised homo-phobia was real. I didn't have it for anyone else; I truly believed everyone should be able to love who they love, but to myself I was a total school bully. My inner child didn't think she deserved to be loved the way other people did. To begin with, I was so uncomfortable in my skin. I was really scared. Why couldn't I just be 'normal?' (a concept that doesn't exist– I may as well have been asking to be a leprechaun). Why did I have to be in a career where opportunities get taken off you, if you openly identify as something – even as casting directors say they are searching for 'authenticity'? If I came out, could I still play straight girls? Something I've made my entire career out of? What if I lost everything? What would people say? Would people look at me differently? Would my friends judge me? These questions might seem overly dramatic to some, but they were a daily battle for me and swam around my head each night. I knew I was utterly miserable hiding part of myself. I was desperate for connection, something all humans are hardwired for, but I couldn't take the leap. It's weird to navigate an industry that publicly celebrates difference and authenticity, but also gave me zero representation of famous, lesbian actors. Mainly due to so few roles that centre LGBTQIA+ identities.

It's about what feels right for you

Eventually, like a pot about to boil over and ruin your stove top, you have to make a choice. Stay silent in the closet and get on with your life miserably, while fantasising about marrying Emma Stone in secret, or take a risk and jump into a new life. As you stand at the crossroads, how do you know which way to go? I like to think the world rewards courage, and coming out takes heaps of it – no matter what others might say. Sure, for those people who've been brought up in an environment of total safety and acceptance, coming out may not feel like a huge issue – but that is not the case for most. It is a *big* deal, no matter how liberal we like to think our society has become, and there is no right or wrong way to do it. It's totally your decision how you play it. Do you want a gender-reveal-style video where you cut the cake and show off its rainbow layers? Go for it, girl! Do you want to tell just a few close friends and let the news spread naturally through the update channel of society? Equally as fabulous. Or do you just want to write it on a piece of paper and hand it to one trusted friend? You'll know what feels right for you.

No matter how you approach it, there will always be people who'll talk behind your back, because some people simply have nothing better to do and think it connects them with others (no true connection has ever been formed through gossip, despite what *Sex and The City* might have you believe). This is why other people have to be irrelevant in this decision – it's all about you, baby. I say that with hindsight, because at the time I didn't want people's perception of me to change and I was so worried what people were going to think. I kept myself in chains because I was too worried about other people, rather than myself. I am exactly the same person, no matter who I date. Other people will never define me. I still obsess over Taylor Swift's every move, eat far too many cookies, and forget to pay my water bill every month, but instead of a man not being able to take a shower at my apartment, it's a woman.

I was concerned people wouldn't take me seriously. Was I sure? Was I GOING THROUGH A PHASE? Was it just like when I attempted to be Avril Lavigne all over again? (I'm not kidding: we're talking many months during my teenage years.) Or was I just simply exploring my sexuality like every young woman should? I don't know what boxes I thought I had to tick to be considered a 'legitimate lesbian', but I was scared of failing. Was it like the test you have to take to become a British citizen? And what about the men I'd dated previously? What would they think? (Why did I care?) I had this faux responsibility that they'd be worried they'd turned me gay in some way and it would ruin their self-esteem. As a certified people pleaser, I was more worried about them!

In a moment of feeling totally lost and unable to decide what to do, I asked the universe for some direction. Literally like a mad woman, I spoke to the clouds as I ambled down the road. I was on the way to babysit for a family I adored, and as the rain pelted down, I genuinely shouted to the sky for help. When I arrived at the house, I was ushered into the lounge and told to shut the door. I remember thinking, 'Oh they're defo getting a divorce.' Instead, the mum sat me down and told me she'd been diagnosed with cancer. My jaw hit the floor. Here she was, two young children, a great job and a gorgeous house. All the things we're taught to want growing up – the things that are the goal, the coveted pillars that, once achieved, will support our happy/ normal/functioning/[insert positive adjective here] life.

Then she told me I had to live life for me, I had to do all the things I wanted to because none of us know how much time we've been granted. I needed that push, I think, to embrace living for me, not for anyone else – and not to feel guided by those notions of what I should be doing. So many of us conduct our lives in a certain way to appease our parents or families. But as adults, we don't need that connection to them in the same way as when we were little kids. We no longer depend on them for our survival. We can live our lives for us. In a way this can be a really difficult truth to accept; we may not *need* our connection in the same way, but we might still *want* it nonetheless, which can complicate things.

I'm not suggesting we all become insane narcissists who don't consider anyone else's feelings, but when it comes to your sexuality, that is yours. We only have one chance (that we know of) on this earth and I didn't want to spend it in a miserable, dark closet. I didn't want to imagine the rest of my life denying this part of myself.

Many of us delay coming out. A recent study showed girls in their twenties are the most likely to delay because being a lesbian is seen as 'over-sexualised' 'masculine or butch', 'cringey or awkward' 'unattractive' and 'man-hating'. A third of lesbians also said they delayed coming out because being a lesbian is seen as 'wrong' and is viewed as 'taboo'. Let's get it straight (the only thing in this book): those words and thoughts are perpetuated by heterosexual people who don't get it . . . and that can make you feel shame . . . but no gay girly is making statements like that.

So, what's next? Like I said, first, you have to come out to yourself. That's not me suggesting you throw a lonely party for yourself and three cats with a cake that has 'Congrats you're gay!' iced on it. You might be thinking, girl, I know I'm gay, how can I tell myself something I already know? What do I do? Say it three times in a mirror and Clare Balding appears? Well, it's all about acceptance. You can know something to be true, but transitioning that knowledge to feeling it in your bones is a whole other thing. If you're hiding or denying your truth from yourself, it's going to be hard to truly connect with others. They're not meeting all of you – just a version, a mask. And it might be time to take off that mask. There's some truth in the idea of 'How can others accept you if you don't fully accept yourself first?' I had to be OK with being gay. I couldn't keep pushing the fact back into the imaginary wardrobe in my head where I put things I don't want to think about (I know, literally putting myself in the closet). I had to fling back the doors of that antique, wooden cupboard and sit with all my thoughts and feelings around being gay.

And it wasn't a process I completed in a day. Even a week. And yes, I was very lucky I had help. Essentially, I had to do what many therapists refer to as 'The Work' and unpick why I was the way I was to throw the false beliefs I had out the window and rewrite my narrative. I had to be OK with being gay.

A list of who not to listen to

I know we're here again, but this bit is important, so apologies for sounding like a stuck record. Who had told me it wasn't OK to be gay? Well, there's a few that make that list:

Society. A bleak scroll of X on a bad day would have me under the duvet quicker than a dose of melatonin. I'm still haunted by the story of the two girls who were brutally attacked on the top of a double-decker bus just because they were openly out. If people could stop beating us up, that sure would be great. I can't afford self-defence classes, and I have the upper body strength of a mouse. If someone attacks me, I will just have to lie down on the pavement and ask them to make it quick. Society doesn't go out of its way to make us feel safe, even if it is the minority committing these heinous crimes.

Religion. Mum's twice-yearly jaunts to church at Easter and Christmas apparently qualify her as a card-carrying Christian. And from sitting through those freezing services, wondering how Jesus got his hair to stay so luscious and frizz-free in that heat with no access to a serum or conditioner, it was clear the church wasn't a massive fan of me. Although there are LGBTQIA+ churches cropping up slowly, I'm not a fan of any religion, especially one where a man (Henry VIII) couldn't keep his dick in his pants and be a loyal husband, so created a whole new branch of the religion just so he wouldn't get in trouble for getting a divorce. Like a four-year-old making up their own rules to their own game! And don't get me started on the many religions where it's literally a sin to be gay or you'll be cast out, set on fire, thrown over a cliff or eaten by great white sharks, all to a soundtrack of The Cheeky Girls (artistic licence, but you get the gist). How can you judge someone for who they love based on scripts written thousands of years ago? That have absolutely been edited? And are often wilfully misinterpreted by people who are trying to prove a point? Google Apocrypha and buckle in, kids, we're talking decapitation, Nephilim, possession and magic (George R. R. Martin, eat your heart out).

Finally, TV and films offering zero representation – except the odd lesbian best friend as a side part – meant I had no one to relate to while I was growing up. I didn't want my life to be a plot device for the heterosexual people, thank you very much. Or the B character who gets killed the second they find love and happiness. So, I was going to have to take ownership of my sexuality knowing that prejudice exists in all walks of life, and that many people would rather judge and gossip than have a conversation and educate themselves. At the root of most homophobia is fear. People fear things they don't understand (or don't want to understand), and parents pass on their beliefs to their children like shitty traditions. Most of our fears come from our parents, and I realised I actually don't care if Chris down the road and his parents are massive homophobes, I'll just take them off the Christmas card list.

Before coming out, though, I knew I wanted to go on a date. Not to make sure I was definitely making the right decision (my time in Europe had told me what I needed to know about my sexuality), but I felt I needed a test drive. Like I needed to have been on a date before I could say anything. A badge of legitimacy, if you like – which I now know is utter bullshit. You do not need another person to confirm how legitimate your sexuality is, but I was a naive baby gay at this point. There was just one problem . . . as a 'passing heterosexual' I didn't actually know that many gay women. I had more gay men in my life than straight ones – but the lesbian/gay men Venn diagram doesn't really have all that much crossover, and I wasn't part of a fun, queer community yet. I saw women on Instagram, living their excellently clothed lives in Hackney . . . but how to infiltrate? Hackney was a trek on the Overground, and I had (still have) the fashion sense of a toddler who got dressed in the dark. How do you get your first same-sex date? Is it legal to advertise that on Instagram? 'WANTED: A female to date me. Over thirty cos hashtag Mummy issues, must enjoy cake and cats.' Surely that wasn't asking for much?

I didn't quite have the confidence for dating apps, and meeting new people brings me out in hives. I would rather be hit by a lorry than walk into a room full of people I don't know. How was I going to do this? Enter the two lesbians I did know, my best friend Jess and her ex, Becca. They put the word out in what I like to think of as the lesbian WhatsApp group chat of London, and another of Becca's exes came forth and showed interest in an exchange I can only assume was like someone adopting a dog from Battersea. Do all lesbians of London date each other in an incestuous circle of heartbreak? I'm suspecting so. Enter Rachel, as we'll call her – she had seen photos of me after a little Instagram stalking and asked Becca for my number. She was over thirty, liked cakes and dogs, but I reckoned I could twist her arm to my feline friends. We arranged to meet for a drink, and being the most indecisive person on the planet, I let her choose the place. I don't really drink alcohol (the last time I drank three martinis I ended up in a relationship with a man which did so much damage that my therapist can afford a new extension), but I always wait to tell people face to face as it's a good green/red flag indicator. The day rolled around, what to wear? Jeans and a nice top? It's jeans and a nice top, right? It's always jeans and a nice top.

We meet outside the *Harry Potter* theatre in London (yes, I know it's not called that, but you knew exactly where I meant when I said that, so don't be a dick). She's over 6 foot, and for context I'm 5 foot 2, and already enjoying the natural comedy of this. So many jokes to be had. She leads me to a small road in Soho where we stop and stand in front of a black door that reads 'SEX SHOWS DOWNSTAIRS'. My heart lunges so hard and fast I'm surprised it doesn't break my ribs. When I said I was 'chill with going anywhere', I meant an All Bar One or a Spoons, not a lap dance on the first date. I'm not against places like these as long as everything is consensual and the performers are happy, but I'm as British as they come and I'm trying to quell the rising panic in my throat. How can I make an emergency exit? Collapse on the floor? Bolt and leg it down the street, block her number and die from embarrassment? I can feel myself becoming irrationally angry at Becca. Has she set me up with a sex pest? Is that even a thing with women? Why are there beads of sweat dribbling down my back? I don't have time to weigh up my options before I'm ushered into a dimly lit corridor where paintings of naked girls and men in gimp masks adorn the walls, and there's a giant sign saying 'Spankings £10' – along with the level of harshness you can ask for – looming over the reservation desk.

'What can I do for you?' the hostess asks. 'We're just here for a drink,' replies Rachel, and the elastic band around my chest releases slightly. OK, maybe we can just have one drink and I'll avert my eyes to the floor and try not to act like a twelve-year-old who finds all this totally mortifying. 'Head right down' the hostess gestures and Rachel ushers me to go first. Clearly my people-pleasing tendencies have returned in full fashion, as I tiptoe down the stairs imagining what sight is going to greet me. But when I push back the curtain, to my utter surprise, I'm met by a small bodega. It's just a wine bar, filled with fully clothed everyday humans, and zero naked dancers. I clearly can't hide the relief on my face as Rachel laughs, 'Oh the sex stuff? It's just a gimmick, did it scare you?' (No shit, Sherlock, I was about to have an aneurysm.) We find ourselves a small table towards the back. We have great conversation on how we both found our sexuality. She was previously married to a man for a visa and hated it, I secretly obsessed over older actresses I fancied. Was I panicking most of the time? Yes. Did my heart rate slow down? A bit. But did I fancy her? Not really. It felt like a chat between mates, rather than chemistry. And that's OK.

We had one more drink and said our goodbyes. Neither of us texted each other so I guess we both felt the same way. Not ghosting per se, just nonchalant. But I wasn't disappointed. Quite the opposite: I felt proud, which was usually an emotion that made me deeply uncomfortable. I had the shiny badge of giving it a go – I put myself out there and it wasn't quite right, but I was sending a message to the universe that I was ready for this. Raising my vibration, if you're into that sort of thing. The date confirmed that I was on the right track and gave my overly anxious brain evidence that this was the path for me.

Once I felt solid enough in myself on my newly found Rainbow Brick Road, I thought I had better tell others, so I decided to test the water amongst friends. On my birthday night out at a roof-top restaurant, a TikTokker (yes, I know it's a bit cringe, but my nightly scrolls help me sleep, despite what medical advice suggests) who I find very funny and attractive sashayed across the floor. I turned to my mates and with the courage of my once-a-year-birthday-porn-star martini inside me, I gasped, 'I fancy her *soooo* much.' Cue a brief moment of silence, before everyone burst out laughing. This opened the conversation up to questions about other women I fancied, and no one threw me off the roof. Result!

Over the next year or so I slowly dropped in hints and phrases amongst coffees and lunches and casual conversations, and to my surprise most people didn't even flinch. I even got a couple of 'OMG I KNEW IT!'s – clearly, I was not as subtle as I had thought. I drip-fed it, until everyone close to me knew. I never came out to my parents (no doubt an important or scary event for some), I just let the message find its way to them through my sister or snippets of conversations. I was lucky that whatever their reaction was going to be – I decided I didn't care. I personally didn't feel the need to have a big social media announcement at the time, but if that's what you fancy, you do you, babe, live your best life, get that rainbow sexuality reveal cake!

Recently, I was working on a job where I told two men I was gay. The first one, we'll call him Simon, has been in a long-term relationship with his same-sex partner for eleven years. When discussing dating, I slipped in that my pool of choice is slightly more limited because my Hinge is well and truly set to women, and the biggest, most genuine smile spread across his face. There was a moment of connection, an 'I get you, babe'. It's not that either of us made a fuss about it, it was just that in that moment, I knew he understood.

The next, let's call him Liam, was a drop-dead gorgeous actor. Once, we had a scene where he confessed his undying love to me, and he almost made me believe I was straight. Almost. We'd spent a couple of days together and really hit it off – but when I mentioned that it was girls I fancied, it was like he didn't know how to react! What to do with his face! How would he categorise me? Suddenly, it seemed as though I didn't fit into his stereotypes of women. He was so taken aback that part of me believes he hadn't met a lesbian before. He maybe thought we were imaginary, like unicorns, or thought all 'lesbians' must like men really if they only met the right one, kind of like the Archbishop of Canterbury thinking he can make a man king by placing his hand on his head. Or there was the time I told a male friend I was gay, and he suddenly started calling me 'Mate', having never done so before.

My favourite experience of coming out was with my best mate Fraser. We'd met outside a particularly dry English literature class on our first week of sixth form, and out of a line full of girls he strode towards me and introduced himself. Today they identify as gay and non-binary, but at the time they were the loveliest boy in an array of floral shirts who spent all their lunch times flinging themselves around in the dance studio. We were inseparable to the point of most people thinking we were dating. We weren't, but at seventeen we made a pact that if we weren't married by forty, we would marry each other, and even drew up a list of baby names: Dulcie, Woody, Elsie, Willow – vaguely Victorian and genteel seemed to be our brief. Every so often someone would ask me if Fraser identified as straight. Admittedly we did spend a lot of time singing along to the *Wicked* soundtrack – I would reply I didn't know, as Fraser had never raised it with me, and we were just us. But when the big reveal came a year after they'd left for dance school, of them and their beautiful new boyfriend, I was delighted. Cut to me, all these years later munching through a chicken burger telling them I was now solely dating women, and yes, I too was gay and trying not to choke on a bit of lettuce when they erupted in squeals of glee. We couldn't help but laugh at the fact we spent our teenage years being each other's beards. I like to think we pulled it off, but our peers might dispute this fact, and I still have hopes of our mousy-haired children when I need a sperm donor – maybe those baby names will come in useful!

Of course there were the common annoying phrases that most people get thrown their way once they come out.

- How did you not know? (Poor vision. I got glasses.)

- You don't look gay. (And you look straight?)

- What's it like? (It's like eating food your entire life
  and then someone introducing salt and pepper and
  spices, and you're like, 'OMG this is what food is meant
  to taste like!')

- I would never have known! (OK, Miss Marple.)

- Did you not like being with men? (I thought we were all
  just closing our eyes and waiting for it to be over?)

- You just haven't found the right man yet. (Have you?
  Where are the good ones? Costco?)

- And my personal favourite: I bet I could turn you
  straight! (Sure, give it a go, lad!)

But I am well aware of my privileged experience of having a supportive reaction to coming out. That's not the case for everyone.
I knew my grandad, for example, would cut me off. A retired
ex-army eighty-year-old, I remember as a young teenager watching Rihanna perform on *The X Factor* and making the comment
that she was, 'OMG so hot' (truth) and being told if I was ever
gay, I wouldn't be welcome in his house. Look, Manchester
takes ages to get to and I can live without the annual birthday
tenner from him. It's his loss.

But some people live with the threat of being cut off by
their friends and family for being gay, for all sorts of (inherently
wrong) reasons. It's totally normal to fear rejection from the
people you love. No one wants to be alone. But as an adult, we
can handle that rejection if it does occur, and we need to try to

make decisions that benefit us. If they can't accept you as you, they don't love you, no matter what they might protest, and there will be plenty of people you might not have even met yet who will love you just the way you are (Bruno Mars wasn't lying). In the words of Taylor Swift anyone who doesn't accept you, really needs to calm down.

Sometimes coming out doesn't exactly go to plan and people react badly. Hearing any news that is different from a person's expectations can initially cause a dramatic reaction. Our brains naturally react to surprising news with denial and anger far quicker than they are able to react with total acceptance and love. But often initial reactions are just that, and they can change over time. The first time you hear a song you might not be into it, but after a week it's the only thing you've got playing. Sometimes people need time to come round to things, but it's not your something you should have to worry about. There are many people who have to come out many times in order to really get their family and friends to see them as they are and be validated, but at the end of the day you are worthy of feeling validated as a human being, no matter what human being you are and whoever you love.

I think it's a decision where you have to choose you, over everyone else. Like the inner child healing. If you were sitting with your six-year-old self, and you had to pick between looking after them, or appeasing a bunch of adults (who, let's face it, should know better than to inflict their views on others), you'd protect that child, every time. And that little girl lives inside you still and needs your support and compassion to help guide her through life. She needs to know that you'll be on her side, no matter what. Once you've come out, don't be afraid to bring up your sexuality. Think how much your friends talk about the guys they fancy and are dating – you're allowed the same experience as them. If it feels awkward that's on them, not you. It's wonderful to be able to talk about sexuality in an open way.

That being said, it also doesn't have to be something that defines you; you get to set the parameters of what it means. Sometimes you have to find yourself coming out every day, to the hotel receptionist who's trying to put you and your girlfriend in twin beds, to the doctor who assumes 'sexually active' means you're dating a man, to holding your partner's hand in public. While it would be handy to whack everyone in a WhatsApp group chat and make sure they've all read it, the world isn't quite there yet.

Very few people regret coming out, and most report wishing they had done it sooner. An elderly gentleman in New York came out at eighty-two because he realised he didn't have long left, and he'd spent all of his life hiding his identity and didn't want to pass away with that regret. So he went out to a pride party and nabbed himself a toy boy boyfriend. I think we could all learn something from him. When I came out, I genuinely did feel lighter . . . younger, almost? The liberation that comes with being your authentic self is huge. The relief of not having to hide a part of yourself any more. Even if it's not something you think about every day, sexuality is a big part of our lives, and we can't just ignore it like a parking ticket and hope it will go away. If you ignore it, it will cost you more in the long run!

It does take courage, there's no denying that. But you have that in bucket loads. Once we strip away the layers of agendas, thoughts and opinions that have squashed our true selves, we have space to just be, to live, exactly as we are.

PART THREE

GO!

11

Lesbihonest

Dear Diary,

My friend says my walls are very high and made from steel . . . and goddammit, I think she might be right. I am the Great Wall of China. There is nothing more terrifying to me than dating.

It's not that I don't like people. I love people! Just at arm's length – in a 'Please don't come too close and please don't hurt me' sort of way. Like let's have a coffee and put the world to rights for an hour but you're not coming home to watch Gilmore Girls *with me. More importantly, what if I fall for a girl who doesn't like cats or, worse, is allergic? I've already dumped my sister because of this. If she wants to see me, she just has to stare through my living room window. Are my three feline babies getting in the way of intimacy? There's no room on my bed for anyone else. Molly Moon will not give up her pillow for a stranger. And if they don't like Taylor Swift, what are we going to talk about? How on earth am I going to be able to date like this? I have an avoidant attachment style except for maybe three people who I adore, and I'm so anxiously attached to them that I have to check they're alive by checking their Instagram every day. But everyone else I hide from. Chief ghoster. I just can't be relational.*

OK. I know. I'm making up every excuse in the world to not start dating again. Men are from hell and women are from heaven, that's how it goes, right? If not, I fixed it!!

The main pro of now dating women is that I'm statistically way less likely to be murdered if I go on a date. I mean I'm sure there are many pros, but not dying seems to be a key one. I love the idea of having a date and not getting kidnapped at the end of it, as well as not having to send my locations to my friends, tell them where I'm meeting and send appropriate social media accounts to them in case the data needs to be tracked. God, the checklist of being a woman is exhausting sometimes. As if the female load that we get paid 14 per cent less wasn't hard enough, we constantly have to think about how to stay alive when we just want to meet someone for a drink!

How do I know if a woman wants to go on a date with me? I could always tell if a guy fancied me . . . is it the same for girls? I don't know how to flirt. My idea of flirting is trying to wink and looking like I've had a stroke in the process or biting my lip so hard in an attempt to look cute that I end up making it bleed.

I've never really dated. In the past I've just been set up with people (I really should bill my friends for the damage), so how is this tiny ginger going to manage it?

Love,
Rosie x

Let's be honest, it can be stressful meeting new people. I'm trying to pretend that I'm not a ten-year-old in a trench coat who's thinking about skincare or death, while trying to decipher if the person across from me not just likes me, but likes me, likes me.

One of the hardest things for me to figure out, when breaking into the land of dating women, was how can you tell when a woman is flirting with you. I wasn't exactly the best at spotting when men were flirting with me, but that still seemed slightly easier. That said, my ability to spot anything is dire . . . If I can't find something I just assume that it's gone forever, even though I often find it five minutes later, right in front of me. The same goes for dating. But with women, I sort of assume everyone wants to be just mates with me. Sure, I'll think 'We got on great', but I get on great with lots of women – the banter is quick, the conversation is playful, I enjoy their company. So how can you tell if there's something more there? How do you know if a woman fancies you?

I got advice from my friend Jess, who said, 'Just go for it, babe. Jump right in.' If that's something you feel like you're ready to do, jump right in! But that required a bit too much bravery for my liking, so I had to find my own way through the battlefield. How do you cross no-man's-land (see what I did there) to make it into the sea of women? Being a newbie was much harder than I'd bargained for and I had no idea how to do it. If you've had experience dating men, there are things they do that just make it obvious they like you: telling you you're hot, saying how fit you look, laughing at your jokes – the problem is that these are all things straight women do, just to be nice. One of the things that makes it difficult to tell if a woman fancies you is you don't have outward signs like rutting male behaviour (like when a bull stomps its foot, or a guy looks down your top).

So here are some little things I've picked up that may help you decipher if she's really just that into you.

- The most obvious hack to tell if a woman is into you is how she compliments you. A friend will comment on the thing you're doing or wearing, so she'll say, 'I love your top – it looks amazing'. However, gay flirting will focus on the woman not the object – 'You look amazing in that top' or 'You look stunning with that lipstick'. It's all about you.

- They mimic your body language. This might sound creepy, but it's often a subconscious thing we do to make people feel comfortable and to like us. If she's mimicking your movements it's a sign she wants those things for you.

- Laughing – there'll be a whole lot of laughing. (*With* you, I might add, not *at* you.)

- Liking your Instagram stories. (And yes, I know you're checking them to see if she has.)

- Messaging a lot, checking in and finding reasons to have contact. If she's taking lots of opportunities to hang out with you, without stating the bleeding obvious, it's a good sign.

- Lip biting (a bit cringe, but go with it).

- Remembering little things you say. If she brings up little details that you've told her in stories, it's a great sign she really wants to get to know you.

- Initiating physical touch. Hugs, hands on arms . . . you know the drill.

While this isn't an exact science – and good friends might check a lot of these boxes – if there's someone who's doing a combination of all these things, the chances are they may like you, like you. Even if you're not 100 per cent sure, there's no harm in going with it and seeing where it takes you. Sometimes you might read the signals wrong and that's OK too! Trust the process, as they say.

But if a woman hasn't just wandered into our lives and started flirting with us magically, how do we stick our neck out into this wild terrain we know very little about? If, like me, you didn't have many queer female friends you'll probably find yourself navigating the apps. Apps are a good way to establish that you fancy each other, and they do the initial heavy lifting. If your chat turns into an invitation to meet, then great, you know that there's already goodwill there! The queer community are a kind bunch; there's a sort of innate understanding that we've all been on this journey of self-discovery together and that it's not always been easy. A key thing to remember when you start dating is that you'll begin to realise that if you live in a big city, most queer women know each other. My friend Jess was once sat at a table in a bar with her current girlfriend, ex-girlfriend and her ex-ex-girlfriend, who had started dating. It's somewhat incestuous – and a wonderful incentive never to treat anyone badly.

The trickier situation with dating girls on apps is that the idea that men make the first move is ingrained in us. For me, this meant that a lot of liking and matching was done that never crossed over into anything more. There was a level of confidence (and good opening lines) I had to learn before I felt brave enough to put myself out there with a message, let alone go on a date. And what do you do when you don't have much chat? Are girls' pick-up lines as cringeworthy as guys'? My first conversation became a chat about how long our mothers could talk down the phone at us (I can put her on speaker, straighten my hair and tidy my flat). We then agreed to set both of them up on a play date, instead of ourselves.

OK. So part of me was like, do I just launch myself at a girl and hope it works? Initially the idea of a first kiss with a woman seemed like an impossibility. I got lucky, because my first kiss with a girl was actually on screen in a film about two Land Girls who got together while their partners were away fighting in the Second World War. Tragically both husbands survived and returned home and our love had to end. Now, I've done my fair share of kissing and sex scenes in my time. The moment I turned sixteen I was kissing a stranger in a car park in the pissing rain on a night shoot for an ITV drama because that was deemed acceptable. They literally paraded me up and down a line of supporting artists and asked which man I wanted to kiss in the scene. As a teenage girl I didn't have the confidence to say none of them thank you, so picked the one with the kindest face. Anyway, kissing scenes and sex scenes are never sexy. They're choreographed, last hours (see? not realistic at all) and are not particularly fun for anyone involved. Usually when I watch them back, I have to hide behind a pillow because I think I look so awkward. Like I'm copying how to make out with someone. That included a sex scene I did with a very famous actor before I'd even had sex in real life. I just laid there, head on the pillow, facing the wall and barely moving as he thrusted behind me. Unsurprisingly it was the least sexy scene you could imagine. But that wasn't the case for my first on-screen kiss with a woman.

Like something out of a John Lewis Christmas ad, as 1930s' music plays over the wireless, I turn up on my lover's doorstep as she's decorating the tree. As I walk into the lounge adorned with tinsel, paper chain angels and a roaring fire, I lift mistletoe above my head and she kisses me. There are moments as an actor when the crew melts away. When the cameras aren't there. This was one of them. When I watched this kiss back, I was in awe. It was soft, romantic, gentle . . . it felt real. There was nothing salacious or gratuitous about it. And more importantly, it looked like I loved it. Because . . . I did.

I just needed to work out how to take that from on screen into real life. I knew if I could do that, my life (and kissing) would be so much better.

And I was correct. There are so many wonderful perks to dating women: congratulations if your style is similar, as your wardrobe may have just doubled in size! You can have conversations feeling like, on some cellular level, the other person might just get it! There's an innate understanding of what it is to be female! You don't have to overexplain your emotions and you don't have to worry about getting accidentally pregnant. You do however sometimes have to explain to the doctor that yes, you are sexually active, but no you cannot possibly be pregnant, and the doctor still can't work out how that's possible. Or when you go on holiday, the receptionist gives you a twin room because she thinks you're having a girls' holiday away! Society hasn't quite caught up yet!

But with all relationships there are some trickier things too. Think balance.

As women who have relationships with other women, we are basically the emotional equivalent of raging Taylor Swift fans taking down Jake Gyllenhaal. I can only imagine the chaos if your hormones sync on the same cycle. (Although hiding under a duvet hysterically crying into ice cream together does sound great.) I've also heard a lot about overthinking, trying to assume what your partner might be feeling because you're wired similarly (it doesn't mean you're a mind reader), and your identities blending due to your similarities, which could all cause friction. But don't let me put you off. You can do this!

Getting back into the dating saddle

So how do we ask someone out? Look, we have to put ourselves out there. The worst thing they'll say is no and the world won't explode – your ego might be bruised, but you'll survive. Better to try to establish connection than stay safe and walled. A rejection is just redirection! A lot of girls worry about asking someone out who may not be gay. A friend once said to me, 'But how can you tell who's a lesbian to begin with?' (to be fair, a valid point that I battled with too). I replied, 'Well, how can you tell anyone's sexuality just by looking at them without making assumptions?', and as the famous quote goes, if you *assume* you make an *ass* out of *u* and *me*. Most girls are lovely and would be flattered to be asked out, and not offended. They may just correct you and tell you they're not into girls. If that's the case you can just reply with:

'I read that wrong, I'm sorry. You're beautiful – have a great day!'

Every single person, even if not in a romantic sense, has been rejected at some point. It's part of life. Flirting with women is not rocket science, it's just a vibe of whatever comes naturally to you. Don't imagine how hard it's going to be to ask someone out – imagine the discomfort of never doing it.

The queer community is terribly online, so if you're looking to explore away from the apps, please come hang out on QueerTok (the LGBTQIA+ creators on TikTok). You'll find a whole community of women supporting each other.

If you've never dated a girl before (or maybe never dated anyone), you might wonder: is it really so different from dating a man, or is dating just dating? Society has given us rigid structures of what 'men' and 'women' are, but it's a cliché to tar all men with the same brush, just as it is to think that dating women is just all cuddles and talking about your feelings. Society has fed us very distinct and, in some ways, discrete ideas of male and female behaviour as if men and women exist in some sort of vacuum with absolutely no crossover. Which of course is not the case in reality. I'd rather focus on what makes a good date rather than whittle it down to stereotypes. Let's face it, dating is weird. It's like interviewing someone with the view to . . . forever? As someone avoidant (in attachment style and life), whose nickname is 'Little Ghost' (from my ability to run away), I find it quite frankly terrifying. I'm meant to have a drink with someone and know whether when I'm eighty they'll put me in a nice care home? NO THANK YOU. I'm told I'm being dramatic, and that a date is just a chance to get to know someone. You get to meet and see if you gel, and the power either to stay or walk away always lies with you.

If there was any piece of advice I'd give my younger self it would be the permission to leave situations where she was uncomfortable or wasn't enjoying herself. No explanation needed, just get up and walk out. Life's too short and you're allowed to walk away. But when it comes to dating, you do actually have to try.

So you've agreed to go on a date...

Now what makes a good date? It's normal for you to feel awkward or nervous – it's always nerve-wracking when it comes to establishing a connection with someone because it requires a whole load of vulnerability. It doesn't mean you don't like girls or your date!! My biggest fear was what if I've made a mistake? What if I want to run away? I'm terrified of dating, so I've written a list of my top tips.

1   Be upfront about where you're at. Everyone is coming to dating from a different place. At the start of a relationship you have nothing to lose. And there's a lot of goodwill, as there are no stakes. If they can meet you where you're at, great! If not, there are no false expectations.

2   Courtesy and safety are paramount.

3   Dress as you. I was worried I looked too girly on my first date (that goes for your whole queer journey – you're free to dress however you want).

4   Keep it short and have an exit plan in case it's not your vibe. This doesn't stand if you're having a great time and

want to hang out the whole night, but keep an exit plan in your back pocket.

5   Use the date as an opportunity to do something you'd like to try, like pottery painting or a new restaurant. That way if there isn't a connection, you still got to do something you wanted!

6   Activity dates are great as they remove the pressure of having to sit across from each other at a table and answer questions (also a great insight into how someone behaves when they lose!).

7   Be honest. Don't try to force yourself to be something you're not. Show up as you, not as who you think your date might be after.

8   Be curious. Most people love to be asked about themselves.

9   If it's a first date and you're nervous, arrange it at a place where you're comfortable and feel safe.

10   Breathe. Chances are the other person is nervous too. It's OK, be present, be interested and breathe.

11   Don't date someone's potential. Really look at what's in front of you and what's being said.

12   If it's not working, don't try to make it work. It's OK to chalk it up to experience and move on!

13   You can't force chemistry.

Now there is a huge difference between chemistry and compatibility, and for a relationship to work, you need both. So when you're sat at your first date, Merlot in hand, looking at the ceiling as you talk because eye contact is hard (just me?), how do you know there's sparks of romance and not just sparks of enjoying chatting about the latest Netflix blow-up sensation?

I recently asked my Instagram followers what they thought chemistry was, and here are my favourite answers.

- When it feels like you've known them forever and you can be yourself with them.

- When every interaction, good or bad, feels easy and communicative.

- Souls connecting.

- Something we feel on a visceral level. Words often fail that feeling.

- A shared understanding, often unspoken.

- A magnetic pull that makes you want to stay in that person's orbit.

- The undeniable urge to ravish someone.

- The sweet feeling of belonging.

- Physical attraction, intellectual stimulation and humour all combined.

- When a person has shiny eyes and they make your eyes shiny.

- When I understand where the next beat is coming from. Like the comfort of watching a TV programme I love.

It seems to be something that's hard to explain, but it's a reaction we feel in our bodies. Which is a good thing to keep coming back to. How do you feel in your body around them? We are often so cut off from our bodies and living in our heads it's hard for us to check in with how we're feeling, but the body keeps the score and will let us know if something's off. Especially if we dive in too quick, when we might suddenly get that pulling sensation in our stomach or sudden anxiety. We often think butterflies are a good sign, but actually feeling calm and grounded around someone is much better than that sensation of lust and excitement.

A key thing with dating women is just how much we overshare. Do you have actual chemistry, or have you just shared your life stories for four hours so you feel like you've met your soulmate? We can move fast, and that's not always a good thing. It's important to check in with yourself throughout the date and after the initial rush to see where you're at. All good things take time to grow.

Always bring it back to you.

And bad dates are natural. It's very unlikely you're going to meet the love of your life first time round.

For my first dating app experience that spilled over into real life, she suggested we play mini golf. As we played it was becoming apparent that I have the hand–eye coordination of a hammered hen party trying to play beer pong, but I also noticed that she kept looking at me in a slightly strange way. Like she was trying to figure something out. I've had that look a few times. It's when people recognise me but they're not quite sure where from. When that happens I'm usually left reciting my entire CV before they tell me, no, they don't actually own a telly and have never heard of those shows, making me feel like a massive knob. Towards the end of the date I asked her what she was thinking, and she told me she couldn't get over how much I looked like . . . 'Claire Foy? Stacey Dooley?' I answered, my usual doppelgangers. No . . . I looked so much like . . . her sister! Sure enough, she showed me some photos and lo and behold, she was right, there was an undeniable resemblance. I was unsure as to why she'd agreed to go on a date with me when my Hinge photos are very realistic and I'm therefore catfishing no one. But it was no surprise that after our date, I never heard from her again – no one wants to be reminded of incest every time they go to bed!

A question that echoed in my head amongst all of this was what is a healthy way to date? What's right for one person won't be right for another. Some people go on multiple dates a week and love it, others (raises hands) have to be dragged kicking and screaming out into the adult nursery of a bar. How do you balance staying true to you but also being brave enough to put yourself out there? For me it was more about doing something different. Changing the narrative and allowing myself the space to explore what I wanted, but knowing I could run home and dive into a duvet burrito if necessary.

Then there's the other question of getting off together – when you feel the time has come to explore someone else's female terrain, how does it even work? How do you know who to jump down the Jessica Rabbit hole with to begin with? The short answer is you've got to shop around a bit to find out what you like. Think of it like your first grown-up shop in Sainsbury's.

You're not going to like everything. You'll probably spend too much money and you're going to fuck it up by burning something in the oven at some point. (Step away from the hot waxing strips, ladies.) The choice can be overwhelming, and it's going to take some time to figure out what you want. But in this shop, you can try before you buy.

Although an important point that I learnt quickly was: YOU DON'T HAVE TO FANCY EVERYONE.

Something else to be aware of is the term 'gold-star lesbian'. This refers to the OG Lesbians, the Yoda of Lesbians, the Lesbian Dalai Lamas – these are girls who have never been with a man. Unfortunately, sometimes they get treated like a quest by some women. Straight girls who want to try out what it is like to be with a woman will sometimes sleep with a gold-star lesbian to brag about it, or so that they can be taught by them, but actually they're just looking for a relationship like you are.

Most of my mates are girls. I've always been a girl's girl, and the moment I realised I liked women, I was struck by the panic of 'OMG, all my friends are going to think I fancy them now' and 'What if so-and-so doesn't want to share a bed with me any more when we go on holiday? I can't afford my own room in this economy?! We're in a cozzie living crisis, guys!' I was catastrophising, obviously. Turns out just because you're gay, it doesn't mean you aren't allowed to have taste. The same way I didn't fancy every man I knew (very few actually, and usually only the ones that screamed daddy issues), I don't want to bed every woman. While only 3.2 per cent of the UK's population is part of the LGBTQIA+ community, it's not a scarcity mindset where you take whatever you can get. This isn't the Boxing Day sale at Selfridges where you grab anything that looks vaguely alright. You have a right to choose . . . And once you start to like someone you need to build that relationship.

Relationships are so nuanced. Have you ever tried to sit with a friend and figure out their relationship and suddenly you're three hours in and none the wiser as to why they're with said person? Exactly. Relationships are not right or wrong – they just are. And they're full of feeling. They take a hell of a lot of work.

Whichever way you identify, couples' therapists John M. Gottman and Julie Schwartz Gottman have come up with questions to see if you're really compatible in their book *Eight Dates*. These can be used for initial dates or long-term relationships when you want to strengthen your relationship. I've edited them into bitesize questions for you to think about.

Trust

Trust is the foundation of relationships. And although no one is 100 per cent trustworthy all the time, it's the knowledge that someone will value you and be there to support you. To deepen any relationship, we need to understand the other person's beliefs about trust.

How do you define trust? Where do we agree and disagree on issues of trust?

Disagreements

Disagreements in relationships are totally normal and healthy, and managing them even strengthens your relationship. Knowing how your date or partner wants to manage disagreements means that when the time comes you're prepared.

What did you learn about conflict and managing conflict growing up? How would you like to manage conflict in the future?

Sex

A healthy sex life is important to any relationship (even if you're British like me and would rather die in a hole than talk about it). But it looks different for every dating scenario and relationship. It's whatever feels good for both you and your partner. But you have to be honest about what you want. A healthy sex life is rooted in an honest conversation. Research shows that couples who talk about their sex life have better sex more often (Valvano *et al*, 2018).

What do you like? What would you like me to do in our sex life?

Finances

Money is a source of conflict in relationships. Spending habits/saving ambitions/how does any young person afford a house ever again? By being open about your relationship with money you can effectively anticipate and navigate discussions around money and build a healthy financial future together.

What did you learn about money growing up? What makes you anxious about money? What do you hope for your financial future?

Family

For me and for many others, differing visions of a family can be a deal breaker. I've known I've wanted children since I was a toddler whacking my BABY Born around, and I know this might not be for everyone and it's unfair to expect someone to change what they want for you, so it's good to know this before entering into a potentially long-term commitment with someone. Sadly, as women we are time-limited on our ability to conceive naturally, so it's always good to plan ahead.

Ask your partner or date what their dream family would look like.

Fun and adventure

Play is a necessary and vital part of intimate relationships. We often mistakenly think we have to have matching ideas of fun and adventure for the relationship to succeed. Of course, it's great if you do, but it doesn't matter if you don't. You love marathon running and I love making forts out of pillows and hibernating . . . that's totally OK – I can cheer you on from my den! The most important thing is to find as many ways as you can to play together, and then support each other in your separate adventures.

What does play and adventure mean to you? In the last few years what's the most fun you've had?

Spirituality

Spiritual intimacy can allow you to grow closer. Does that mean getting my partner to do affirmations with me every morning, 'I AM ABUNDANT AND HAVE LUCKY GIRL SYNDROME', and meditate to calming music? Not necessarily. But connecting spiritually, even if your views don't align, can still bring you together and create great emotional intimacy.

What rituals can we do together to help strengthen our connection?

Dreams

I love a dream come true. I'm lucky that I've had many experiences that have made me feel like Lizzie McGuire at the end of her Rome adventure singing, 'This is what dreams are made of', but recently I was speaking with other people about our relationships to dreams. Everyone had a really bad experience of them. They hadn't been so fortunate to have my experience. I believe a dream is just a plan in action. And by the end of the discussion I was rallying troops to try and set in motion what we could do to make each person's dream come true. Everyone on this planet deserves at least one of those moments in their life. To ensure that your dreams can be fulfilled (OK, realistic ones – maybe not becoming best friends with Beyoncé) you have to understand what your dreams are. Once you and your partner both know what your personal dreams are, you can share them with each other and start to do little things to work towards them.

What is your biggest dream? What would you like to do in order to take steps to achieve it?

If you've started dating someone and think it could be something more, so it's moving from dinners after work into weekends at hers and heading down the M4 to a long-term relationship, we need to talk about the biggest trope in lesbian history – but one that comes with real caution.

CAUTION: Beware of the U-Haul

There's a classic lesbian joke that goes like this:

> *What do lesbians bring on a second date?*
> *A removal van.*

An 'urge to merge' is a stereotype associated with lesbians as we have a tendency to form very deep emotional connections very quickly. We move in together after a short period of time, start dressing similarly, live in each other's pockets and slowly merge into the same person.

Fusion, merger and enmeshment are terms that have been used in the literature to describe lesbian relationships, and they all apply.

When we fall in love with women, we often find we're so similar that it's easy to lose our identities in each other. (But we've already done identity work in this book, remember? So let's not give up ours for someone else!) We become each other in a really unhelpful, unhealthy way. And this is why lesbian break-ups can feel like you've been split in two.

For decades the 'urge to merge' was the practical thing to do. Back then, if you found a partner you held on to them. A bit like when you had the same partner in netball all year: it's too dangerous to change things up for fear you'd be left without one. In the lesbian world, serial monogamy was safe and rewarding.

And why wouldn't we hold on to a relationship in which we finally feel fulfilled? If we've grown up being told wanting to be with a woman is wrong, but also that relationships are an essential on the checklist, you end up walking an intense tightrope.

Biologically our brains are wired for relationships and connection. Dr Amy Banks, instructor of psychiatry at Harvard Medical School in the USA, says a good example of this is mirror neurons, which are located throughout the brain and help us read other people's feelings and actions. They may be the neurological underpinnings of empathy – when two people are in conversation they are stimulating each other's mirror neuron system. There have been studies that look at human emotions such as disgust, shame and happiness, where the same areas of the brain light up in the listener who is reading the feelings of the person talking. We are, literally, hardwired to connect. As women we usually have higher levels of oxytocin than men. Oxytocin, often known as the 'love drug', is a hormone we release when falling in love, having sex or breastfeeding. It's essentially a biological nod to attach. Since there are two women in a lesbian relationship, there's twice as much oxytocin buzzing around . . . things feel amazing, very quickly.

In order to bypass the U-Haul and move in with someone when you're truly ready, we need to find happiness not just within our relationship, but from a variety of sources: our friendships, our family, our work, from recreational activities we enjoy. Spend time outside the relationship bubble. We all have friends who disappear for six months when they enter a relationship and while it's understandable, it's not always healthy.

We need to look at our relationship in an objective way, which can be hard when you've sunk a love potion and have a million hormones flying about. Is this relationship healthy? Can we communicate? Are we actually compatible or just obsessed with each other? We need to not get sucked into the head rush of getting to know someone, and work on building intimacy and connection. If it's meant to be, it'll still be there once you've laid the solid foundations.

12

What is love?

Dear Diary,

I sit on Hampstead Heath watching couples entwined on the grass, sharing a picnic and drinking champagne out of sticky plastic glasses. Families fly kites as they run down the grassy slopes with their toddlers, laughing, as the mum tries to take photos of these moments that feel precious to witness. Maybe just another Saturday to them, but if I could distil that joy and sell it, those magical moments of heads thrown back, white teeth, laughter and love – I think I'd be a millionaire. And here I am in this vacuum of impossibility. I don't want to eat ready meals alone for the rest of my life, no matter how many cats I can buy to keep me company. My lot think I'm part of their tribe now, and have cajoled the local kittens to turn up on the doorstep to make our pack stronger. I didn't think my twenties would look like this. I was promised Polaroid picture moments and dancing until midnight, not staring at my ceiling at 10 p.m. wondering what everyone else is up to. I stare around my room and think, is this it? Is this really what life is about? I know someone else will not complete me, but we all need connection to survive. I don't want to be one of those babies in that experiment where they

*starved them of love to see what happens. I want to experience the
teen romance, driving with the top down, sort of love. How do I
find it? Or as Oliver sung 'Where-ere-ere-ere is love?' Is it hiding
behind the sofa? Is this what love is? I asked around and got the
following responses:*

'Drive safely.'

Hanging up the wet laundry.

Their hand on your thigh in the car.

Knowing what they'd order on a menu.

Roasting a chicken for you.

Buying and reading books you recommend.

Picking you up after a night out.

Listening to songs you love.

Showing up, no matter what.

Making you a cup of tea.

Finishing each other's sentences.

Running a bath and making sure you get the temperature right.

When icks don't matter.

*Holding each other's baggage and unpacking it together (literally
and metaphorically).*

In London, it's when you travel the distance on the Overground.

Doing the washing up.

Snuggling on the sofa.

It's 'How are you feeling?' after a long day.

'Put your seatbelt on.'

Doing the driving when you're tired.

*Not watching your favourite show without you (or pretending
convincingly they haven't).*

'I saw this meme and thought of you.'
Someone feeling like home?

Love,
Rosie x

Those are the responses to my in-depth research, done very professionally on Instagram, when I asked people what love is to them. While they're all different, they all share a commonality.

The wonderful thing about love is how it shows up in our lives in so many unique ways. The best loving relationships don't need to be categorised neatly. How do we describe something that's been woven into the fabric of being human and over-analysed and portrayed countless times? The dictionary says it's 'an intense feeling of deep affection'. You may not agree with my definitions of what love is, but that's what makes it so hard to describe. We can describe the physiology of the emotion, but even that's up for debate. Is love heart-racing excitement or is it calm stillness? Is it an inner knowing of safety – a space for refuge, for growth, for pain? We all navigate love in different ways. There are also allegedly five love languages that determine the way we show love. They are:

1   Words of affirmation.

2   Quality time.

3   Physical touch.

4   Acts of service.

5   Receiving gifts.

Which is funny, because I think I have three of them (I think it's normal to have more than one). Definitely not the last one for me. Whenever I open presents, I have to do it in another room away from everyone because I don't know what to do with my face.

And we can't just show love to other people. We have to show it to ourselves. It allows us to build a healthy sense of self-esteem, where we are able to hold all of ourself in warm regard. We're all flawed, we all need work, we all need connection and we are all deserving of love.

If you are not in a relationship it doesn't mean you are somehow incomplete. We are often made to feel like we're not whole unless we have another half. This is untrue. Ignore the Hollywood tropes that are dangled in front of us courtesy of the £14.99 Netflix fee – those writers are making up scenarios for themselves to live in to make themselves feel better (I speak from experience, guys . . .).

We don't pursue romantic relationships because they're essential to our happiness but because we choose to give and share our love, in whatever form that may take. As we quote from *Love Actually* every December . . . Love really is all around. You just have to look for it. Even in the face of knowing that we sometimes get our hearts broken or suffer the loss of a loved one, most of us still stand ready to step into a new relationship and open our hearts to more love. And that's pretty brave in my book.

13

Lez get together

Dear Diary,

I've come to the point in my life where I'd like to be in a relationship again. If it sounds like a decision as serious as taking out a mortgage, it's because it feels like it is. Should I go and sit behind a desk in a bleak, greying office and have a grumpy old man with hair growing out his nostrils review me and see if I fit the criteria? Funny? Check! Alright looking? Check! Scared of intimacy? Cue Britain's Got Talent *style 'UHH AHHH' noise. SORRY, ROSIE, YOU HAVE BEEN DECLINED. Your credit score in being relational is too low. Back on to the streets for a lifetime of loneliness.*

I've done it before. I have been in relationships before. I write that as if I'm trying to convince myself of the fact. Though sometimes they feel like a distant nightmare ago. It's just that they blend from the mundane, the sweetest boy who I had to break up with after we travelled to Paris and ran out of things to talk about after he mistakenly thought the Mona Lisa *was painted by Vincent van Gogh, to the absurd, where I cohabited with a man whose calls I regularly had to decline unless I wanted to be faced with a barrage of vitriol.*

Life, like it always does, has changed so much since then. The main reason being that I've changed so much since then. I'm no longer the compliant, sweet girl who renders herself invisible by having no needs or autonomy. I'm a whole, living breathing human. Sometimes I worry I'm a lot to handle, but then I think that pomegranates are amazing and worth the mess and maybe I'm amazing and worth the mess too, ya know? And now, I'd like someone to enjoy my time with. But I'm the one getting in my own way.

Truth is, despite the universe continually showing me otherwise, I'm scared everyone's secretly out to get me. I know that one of the reasons being in a relationship after trauma is difficult is because trauma survivors don't always have a clear understanding of what love should look and feel like. But I've gone from being anxiously attached to being so avoidant, I've developed the habit of ghosting people. If you're reading this and I haven't texted you back, I'm sorry. Self-isolation, consciously or not, is my attempt to limit contact with people because other people still don't always feel safe to be around.

Case in point is parties. My gorgeous friend Ruby collects people like Sylvanian Families, and she kindly tries to integrate her small, shy friend into her friendship groups like a mum encouraging her toddler to play with others. There have been times where I've been introduced and managed to chat and joke and have a lovely time, and yet there are times when she introduces me to people and I literally can't open my mouth. I am mute. It's as if gaffer tape has been taped over my mouth, and even if I've got something to say it's not coming out. Vocal constipation if you like.

Maybe I'm just a vibes girl? A tarot reader did once tell me I'm a lot more psychic than I realise and I definitely made that my personality for a good six months. If I like your vibe – I'm in! I feel like a little tortoise ready to poke its head out into the world of connection.

But I need to know how to be relational to be in a relationship. So just how do I do it? When I find the one, how do I make a relationship work? How do I stay and not run away? And more than that – how do I make a relationship work with a woman?

Love,
Rosie x

After the Kardashians, relationships are probably the most documented thing on this planet. We're overloaded with movies, songs, series, podcasts and books dissecting them, analysing them and trying to unpick what makes a lovable one, a lustful one or one we want to steer clear of. But the simple truth is: relationships take work. Healthy relationships involve trust, honesty and a whole lot of communication and effort from both people. Each person has inherent worth; neither person is more valuable than the other. There's no black or white; relationships are incredibly nuanced and that's what makes them so hard to pin down. A good way to think about a relationship is like an ecosystem (like that big biome down in Cornwall where they cultivated the jungle): we have to work at getting the balance just right in order for it to flourish. But the work isn't tiring, commuting 9 to 5 stuff, it can be life-affirming things: date nights, walks, weekends away, sharing dessert, finding ways to stay curious and excited by your partner. All way more fun than sitting in an office!

When you first find yourself in a queer or lesbian relationship the most important thing is to throw any ideas or expectations out the window. Follow what makes both of you happy and not what you think you should be doing or what you've been told a lesbian relationship should look like. I know I'm repeating this, but it's intentional because it's so important. There are some obvious differences between being in a same-sex relationship and a heterosexual one – in the latter you might stumble over gender norms, whereas when two women are dating you sidestep them completely and get to make the rules yourself and thus the 'load' of life often gets shared more equally.

Bestselling author Brené Brown explains that relationships are never 50:50 all the time. 'It's never 50:50. Ever,' Brown mentions on her podcast. Instead, she and her husband regularly check in by telling each other their levels in terms of 'energy, investment, kindness, patience'. If one of them is at 20 per cent capacity, and the other is at 80, the partner with more energy to give will take on more of the household chores and offer more emotional support. I'd love to try this as long as no one makes me figure out the leftover percentage – maths was never my strong point!

As mentioned above, there are some big differences between being in a lesbian and a heterosexual relationship. Some are amazing: in a lesbian relationship you come at things from the same place. Nobody's career is more important. Nobody is the 'boss' of the relationship. That does not need to be the case for heterosexual relationships either, but throughout history (and as we see the rise of the tradwife again) it can exist. You have unique insight and understanding into each other, simply by sharing that Y gene. Which means there's far less explaining to do, and that is such a time saver! And then there are some not so great ones: for example, there will be blood. So much blood! (But luckily it does mean there's always tampons available.)

And yet sometimes, because you're both women, there's a direct comparison between you and your partner which can be tricky to navigate. There are no 'Well obviously it's easy for him, he's going through life as a man' excuses here. We're on a (relatively) level playing field.

But mostly what I've learnt is that at the end of the day, it's still a relationship. Intimacy and insecurities, support and friction, challenges and celebrations – everything's still there. While there are things that are more difficult about being with a woman, the big things – both good and bad – are universal.

And a universal theme for us all? Baggage! Nobody enters a relationship without baggage. Even if it's your first one. To every relationship we're bringing in what our parents gave us and modelled for us. How your parents treated you is the best indicator of how you're going to show up in the relationship. Our upbringing, memories, traumas and experiences all inform our ability to be in a relationship. And nothing is more inherited than our attachment style.

Discovering your attachment style

When someone says the phrase, 'What's your attachment style?' You might be thinking I dunno, Word doc? PDF? Microsoft Paint (is that still a thing?)? Not quite. Our attachment style is how we attach within relationships.

Attachment is a biological mandate for us to stick together. It starts right back in infancy when it's not safe for us to be alone and we need our attachments to survive. While we don't need to be attached to someone to survive as adults, that thinking is still ingrained within us and often gets in the way. Your childhood is the biggest predictor of how you act in relationships, because your childhood experiences play out in your adult relationships. And if you don't deal with what you've been through, the person you're dating will. On a subconscious level we are all after the same thing: safety. And it's how we go about achieving that in our relationships that shows up in our attachment styles.

Knowing your partner's attachment style can be really useful, especially at the beginning of a new relationship as it can help you navigate communication, discord and repair. Think of it as one of those quizzes you used to do at the back of magazines that tell you how you love – except with more psychological underpinning. (If I like love hearts over gummy bears, I will be a better communicator, right? I mean it's literally written on the sweets.) There's securely attached, the Holy Grail of attachment which we all wish we could be gifted. Unfortunately not all of us have that solid framework that we can work from. Securely attached adults tend to feel safe, stable and more satisfied in their close relationships. While they don't fear being on their own, they usually thrive in close, meaningful relationships. And then there's the majority of us: the insecurely attached peeps.

There are three main subtypes of insecure attachment: anxious, avoidant, disorganised.

1   **Anxiously attached** – the ones who need lots of contact, reassurance, can sometimes feel a lot of jealousy and

generally want to know their partner is there for them at all times.

2 **Avoidant attachment** is what it says on the tin - they're super-independent, self-sufficient and rarely ask for help. These are the sort of people who often go quiet and shut off from connection.

3 And lastly there's **disorganised** - these are people who are consistent and then inconsistent in a relationship. Adults with this style of insecure attachment tend to feel they don't deserve love or closeness in a relationship, which usually stems from fear.

When navigating your first LGBTQIA+ relationship your attachment style can really show up. For example, someone who is anxiously attached and is finally in a relationship they've longed for, having supressed their emotions and needs for years, is going to want to make sure that the relationship isn't going away. Their anxiously attached behaviours – like constantly checking in or asking if their partner loves them – might really play out.

By knowing our partner's attachment style, we can give them what they need. If they're avoidant you can give them space when they need it, or you can offer reassurance if they're anxious. This builds trust within the relationship. Trust takes consistency and proof that you're going to show up for one another no matter what happens. You have to be congruent with what you say and what you do.

As someone who is about as trusting as King Charles is 'down with the kids', I understand how hard it is to develop trust. But if you don't trust your partner, a good question to ask is how much do you trust yourself? No one is trustworthy 100 per cent of the time – it's whether you can trust yourself to handle the emotions if it does go wrong. In relationships, trust isn't a promise to never hurt each other – it's accepting that risk and knowing that if you do hurt each other, you'll come together to heal.

There are things that we know don't serve a good relationship. Relational Life therapist Terry Real has identified five losing strategies for relationships:

1   **Being right.** As he says, 'What do you want more, to be right or to be in a relationship?' Sometimes we get so caught up in what's happening and our version of events that we prioritise that over the relationship. Proving that you're right is combative and can leave your partner feeling disheartened. Lay down the right card and focus on each other.

2   **Controlling your partner.** Very self-explanatory. We all have our own autonomy and you don't get to be in charge of your partner's life just because you're in a relationship.

3   **Unbridled self-expression.** There are people who go through life saying whatever they feel, without thinking about the impact that their words might have on others. They hide this under a veil of 'authenticity' and 'speaking their truth' – but not everything that's in your head needs to come out of your mouth. I'm not saying we should all be walking on eggshells, too scared to speak up, but not everything needs saying. There are times where we

weaponise therapy speak and are so caught up in 'doing what's right for us' that we don't consider other people's feelings in a particular situation.

4 **Retaliation.** When something happens you fight back immediately, without taking time to pause, breathe and figure out the best way forward for you both. In doing this you unconsciously or consciously hurt the other person.

5 **Withdrawal.** Running away from the relationship won't solve whatever is going on within it, and you'll have to come back sooner or later. Love requires us to look at what's in front of us, not to turn away.

But can they handle 'the real me'?

In the early stages of a relationship many of us find it difficult to show up as our true selves. I once went on a first date, acted as maturely and together as possible, only to leave realising that the other woman was going to get the shock of her life if she ever met the real me: a hyperactive millennial with an excellent taste in dungarees. A lot of us are performing either our 'best selves' or what we think the other persons wants or needs, as if we're some sort of mind-reading Houdini (plot twist: you're never right). We are subconsciously assessing how to keep the relationship and attachment. This dynamic of not speaking up and expressing yourself can then play out in the relationship.

A mistake I made was holding on to a lot of past experiences, trying to navigate not bringing them into a new relationship, and not trusting a partner to be able to handle 'the real me'. It takes time, but opening up to your partner and letting them see all the sides of you helps strengthen your connection. I lug that baggage around thinking that everyone's out to get me, even though the universe has repeatedly shown me that's not the case. Oh, you brought me cookies. Laced with what? Poison?

Express what you're thinking and feeling. Notice when you're tiptoeing and avoiding conflict, as it'll come back later down the line if you don't look at it in the moment. If you don't have needs, you don't exist – you render yourself invisible (and not in a cool Harry Potter way). We must stop romanticising the idea of easy-going people. People are not meant to be easy-going: we're supposed to have needs. We're meant to have emotions, thoughts, opinions and boundaries. I lived for twenty-five years not understanding that I had the power to choose what I wanted my life to look like. I'd been set up on a path from the age of four, thrown into the world of acting, and ticked every box along that tumultuous path to success. And I wanted none of it. Many easy-going people have just self-abandoned, because they were taught to prioritise attachments to others over their own self-expression. But when we start to show up authentically we're choosing ourselves and our partner. We're allowed to have boundaries that leave us both protected and connected at the same time. Fights are normal. It's OK to both love and hate your partner sometimes. You can hold more than one feeling at a time.

There is so much research that shows the most thriving relationships are ones where people can repair successfully. And I don't mean repair the IKEA chest of drawers I broke by putting my cat in the top drawer (though the test should be that every couple should build IKEA furniture, and if they survive that mission then they are officially allowed to be in a relationship).

Repairing in a relationship is how you heal and come back together after a rift, disagreement or rupture.

Not all of us were taught how to repair properly or modelled it in a healthy way by our parents so we have no experience to draw on. Have you ever received an apology that goes a little like, 'I'm sorry IF I . . . ' – yup. That's not an apology. If someone says you hurt them, that's their experience and you don't get to tell them you didn't. An apology is, 'I'm very sorry for the way I've hurt you' – an apology is not, 'Let me explain why you should feel differently about what I did.' Got it? Got it! Why don't they teach us how to be relational in school? We might have avoided some world wars, if people could apologise correctly. (Side note: one of the best lessons I ever got in school was how to do a good handshake: firm, eye contact, smile. Whenever I go into a meeting I still think about my music teacher making us practise it.)

Some of the points below might not be right for you and your partner, but they are good starting blocks for repairing when you need to.

- Reminding each other you're on the same team.
- Explaining to your partner how you feel and what could be done differently next time in a calm way.
- Making light of the situation; have a joke about it (but judge the mood carefully on that one).
- Owning your part in the conflict.
- Use 'and' – not 'but'. 'But' cancels out whatever was said before it.

- Validating each other's feelings.
- Apologising appropriately.
- Asking your partner what they need from you in that moment.

It's good to try to repair as early as possible in an argument. Don't be like me and leave everything to the last minute. You don't need to be seconds away from nuclear war before using the fire extinguisher. I used to feel that repairing meant I'd lost the argument, but actually that's not the case. Taking a moment to come back to the part of you that chooses connection over the need to be right is beneficial. Objective reality doesn't exist in a relationship; you'll both have different views and perspectives over events. Repairing is about putting your relationship first and making sure it's your relationship that wins the fight.

Don't let the little moments of discord build up. Find a way to acknowledge ruptures and make repairs. This way you're building solid secure attachment and trust that you are a team in a healthy relationship. If you exist in an ecosystem you want that environment to be as healthy as possible. The most important thing is that you always come back to one another. To a genuine, equal partnership. You're on the same team, in times of love and sometimes through gritted teeth. You're doing this together.

14

Scissor sisters

Dear Diary,

I never liked sex. In fact, if I'm honest, I hated it. I had a great-aunt who once said she didn't see what all the fuss was about (while nibbling her way through a slice of Victoria sponge), and while that was an unexpected thing to hear from a ninety-year-old woman, I couldn't help but secretly agree. To me, sex was associated with one thing and one thing only: pain. And I think that's not spoken about enough, when so many women experience the same thing. But I know now that having sex with the wrong gender probably wasn't helping and, having experienced abuse, why would I want to do something that hurt me? I didn't want to do the Spanish bull-running competition or a round with Mike Tyson, either. My mantra was always 'this is going to hurt' and I did everything I could to avoid it.

The rucksack of shame I was carrying around with me about my history felt so heavy for such a long time. It seemed omnipresent. I didn't want anyone to come anywhere near me, and I certainly didn't want to touch anyone else. I felt tainted, like a faded portrait of yourself you hope no one notices.

I was scared that all my past feelings were going to come back up during sex. I know that trauma is stored in the memory of our bodies, which is why we're often unconscious of what a huge impact an event may have had on us until we have a strong reaction to something else but can't necessarily work out why. We can't put two and two together and when we do we make six. Our brains know they're in a different scenario, but all the emotions are still there, waiting to come out.

Sex is something that's meant to be a source of pleasure, but when it's been weaponised against you, you can end up with huge feelings of shame that you just can't shake.

But I knew, I know, that I have to reclaim that. Pleasure is a birthright that we all deserve. It was taken from me by men, and by society, that teaches women not only to serve men during sex but also not to prioritise their own pleasure at all. I have a friend who bought both her daughters a Magic Wand when they turned sixteen. I remember her telling me and thinking that was iconic. 'I don't want my girls growing up with the same ideas and shame around sex that I had.'

And she's totally right. We don't have to be ashamed of our bodies and the enjoyment we can get from them. BUCKLE UP, GIRLS, we're about to be taught how to do this properly . . . and this time no cucumbers are involved.

Love,
Rosie x

We're expected never to speak about sex. Sex and money are the two topics of conversation that are off-limits. Especially in

British society. They elicit feelings of embarrassment, and God forbid anyone should ever feel uncomfortable! We're taught not to ask questions outside of the tight confines of what's 'allowed'. Luckily there are now hundreds of sex-positive gurus, books and media we can consume. After all, sex is the most natural thing in the world. Without it, we wouldn't be here. We'll talk more about how embodiment relates to sex later, but my hope is for us all to be embodied in all aspects of our being. Our sexuality doesn't just refer to what we do in the bedroom, but how we live out our whole lives. All embodiment really means is being connected to our internal world. Feet on the ground, proper earthy, integrated selves. But we still live in a reality where sexuality is often something to be discussed behind closed doors. However, I like to think that women like Sabrina Carpenter, who expresses her sexuality for herself and for women, is showing us that we can feel comfortable in our own sexuality.

Our sexual expression has long been targeted as a source of shame, guilt and control. Reinforced over time as inappropriate and taboo, with historians erasing the love affairs of prominent women such as Emily Dickinson, Frida Kahlo, Eleanor Roosevelt. Our sexual and sensual nature has a reputation of being dangerous and thus we think we're safer in rejecting it.

We are born as embodied creatures. If you've ever been in a room with a newborn baby, despite their minute size, they are the most powerful thing in the room. Everything revolves around them. They can make people laugh, coo, cry, panic and even run away. Babies know how to listen to their bodies instinctively and communicate with us when something is wrong. However, as we grow we start to feel the weight of society's expectations and we're taught to conform with normative ideas of who we should be and we move away from our intuitive inner guidance. We turn away from our senses and sensory world and start living in our heads, with reasoning so often valued far more than experience. Living in this way means we miss a whole load of information that our body is trying to communicate.

Embodied sexuality is the full expression of your sexuality through your senses, mind, fantasies, heart and presence of being. When we connect to our senses and body, we emanate a radiant confidence and presence. My embodied sexuality means I am fully present in my body. I look to my body for information when things get scary or uncertain, rather than disconnect from it. It's also about enjoying my body – dancing, playing, running, doing yoga, working out, riding a bike – anything physical where I am connecting to my body feels so good and reinforces the pleasure of living as a physical being and not just as a brain in a jar. The idea that life is not happening to you, but as a result of you.

I've never been able to pinpoint what 'sexiness' is, as it's different for everyone, but you know how you can just tell when someone has something about them? Like an undeniably powerful aura that you're drawn to? Quite often that will be someone who's living an embodied life.

We learn to connect with our body through taking the time to stop and listen. This way we can notice what it's saying and work out what it needs. There are many somatic exercises that can be found on social media or online to help you be in your body, and this can include simple things such as wiggling your toes in your shoes when you feel disconnected or planting your feet on the ground, as well as more complex somatic workouts.

Reconnecting with your body

So, let's all spend time getting to know our bodies and what feels great and I'll just pray my mother never picks up this book! Like most things in life, it all starts with good education. But for the majority of us our education started and ended with putting a condom on a cucumber/banana – that, and the fear of God put into us that if we ever had sex we'd get an STI and die, or worse still, get pregnant! And as women we certainly weren't told that you can have a great sex life by yourself, let alone how to discover what brings you pleasure. But you *can* have a great sex life by yourself, and discovering what turns you on and how to feel pleasure alone, will only benefit you once you couple up! Women don't need other people to have fun! That's a fact that society loves to hide from us. Did you know that companies selling female pleasure products aren't allowed to advertise on any social media? But Viagra companies have a free rein? Or my favourite story: Freud believed only an orgasm from penetrative vaginal sex was legitimate, and any other sort of orgasm, such as a clitoral orgasm, meant a woman was developmentally immature. Essentially, it only counts as *real* sex if a man is sticking his penis in you. JOG ON, FREUD!

Sex can also play a role in the denial of our sexuality. 'Spaghetti girl', is essentially a term that means straight until wet. These are girls who think about other females when turned on, but once the urge had been satisfied talk themselves out of the chance of being gay by deciding girls are just really good material for masturbation . . . and then all their internalised homophobia gets in the way. When you're masturbating, you're closer to your true desires and in that moment the barrier separating what you think of as 'right' and 'wrong' comes down in your conscious brain. And it goes right back up, once it's over. It's a really good way of deceiving yourself.

But once you know what you like as an individual, what does that look like when you throw a second vagina in the mix? The key to good sex (straight or gay) is feeling comfortable with your partner and understanding what each person wants. The best way to do this is through being honest and taking things at your own pace. I was about as clued up on sex as I am on Russian politics (but at least my fun button will only make me orgasm instead of initiating nuclear war). I naively thought a penis had to be involved for it to be considered legitimate sex, until my therapist taught me otherwise (while I hid my head in embarrassment in a pillow like a twelve-year-old). That is not the case: oral, fingering, toys, you name it – it counts. Vibrators are a lesbian's best friend.

We need to explore vaginas. Every single one is different in its own unique way, and I highly recommend you look at your own. It sounds mental, but until recently I had no idea what was even down there (it could have had teeth for all I knew). It's important for you to have a healthy sex life with yourself in order for you to be able to explore with others. As my older (genius) friend said to me, 'You gotta learn how to wank, or you'll never be happy!'

But then there's the question of what are we ladies supposed to get off to? We all know there are men who like to fawn over a lesbian relationship: it's one of the most searched for terms on porn sites. In 2021, it was Pornhub's second most-viewed category. I've often wondered why. Maybe because they'd love to join in? Or they know we're off-limits and they'd like to change our minds?

I once had a man tell me, 'You won't be gay once I'm done with you.' It sounded more like a threat, as if I was going to reply: 'Oh yes thank you, fuck the lesbian out of me please!' The audacity! Anyway, I'm not sure the lesbian content on most of these sites is filmed by women? A lot of porn is unregulated, exploitative and misleading. There are healthy, safe porn sites you can pay for, where you know everyone involved is being treated well, consenting and being paid properly. But for most of the videos out there it definitely doesn't seem to be made for the people it's meant to feature – most say watching them gave them next to no knowledge about how one was actually meant to help someone else get off as a woman.

When it comes to porn, 'lesbian sex' is everywhere, but it's never actually for lesbians. For some reason, it's hard to find 'content' where women are having sex with women, only for women. If you're going to show me two women having sex can it please be in an apartment with beautiful interior design; something out of Soho House with some Neom candles and Sabrina Carpenter played on a cello, please? Or at least something that involves a decent conversation and ends in some cuddling. I'm sorry if we want our porn beautifully lit and well shot with a decent plot line. #Aesthetic babe.

I don't want to see women exploited – which is what it can often feel like. I find myself wondering if the women in porn are having a nice time or if it's something they're having to do. If it's the former, I'm chuffed for them, you do you, girl! But if it's the latter, I feel distinctly uncomfortable knowing people are deriving pleasure from women's pain.

Though society thrives on women's pain. Capitalism would collapse if women were happy. Emotional pain. Physical pain that no one, not even doctors, pay attention to. It's like we're gaslighting 50 per cent of the population. And if I were to watch porn, I'd want it to be something where everyone was getting pleasure.

The S word

Reconnecting with your body takes time, but sex is generally thought to be hugely important for the quality of a relationship. Sure, you can improve the quality of the relationship and the sexual relationship won't necessarily improve. But if you improve the quality of the sexual relationship, the quality of the relationship does improve. We need to be connected physically, as well as emotionally. And having conversations with your partner from the get-go about what you like and what you don't like is paramount. When you don't talk about sex with your partner, there's a whole part of them you don't know, and a whole part of you they don't know. Which, as someone who's a bit scared of intimacy, I struggle with. Intimacy = *in to me you see*. You have to let people in.

And that goes both ways. Sometimes when you're first approaching having sex with women, crossing that line is as hard as getting your foot on the career ladder. Sometimes women don't want to be another woman's first time and want the other person to have more experience. I guess it's almost like taking someone's gay virginity and it can feel like a bit of pressure – and nothing kills the erotic more than pressure. Pressure to be good in bed, pressure to orgasm . . . it needs to be thrown out the window. However, a bit like all those job interviews that require you to have four years' experience and two degrees at the age of eighteen – how are you meant to get the experience without having the experience in the first place? What I lack in experience, I make up for in humour and enthusiasm! There's a level of confidence in yourself you have to hold on to while igniting sex. But once you've crossed that line, girl, you're all in!

The crazy thing about dating women is that sometimes they ask what you like in the bedroom. I KNOW, MENTAL. I always thought sex was something that was for men, done to me by men. It was about their pleasure and I'd often check out, and not just emotionally – I'd be driving down the M4 motorway in my mind, literally trying to drive away. I don't even drive, but I was very much in charge of the white van that was hurtling down the motorway towards Bristol.

If someone suddenly gave me options about what I liked and didn't like, I wouldn't know how to respond. I can barely choose what I want to eat when I'm out for dinner! Sex was all about just getting on with it. And I think that's an experience that lots of girls share. We're not taught about our pleasure and what feels good to us, which is really sad. I couldn't ever answer that question because I'd never been asked it or felt like what I wanted mattered.

Communication is important in intimacy. And it's so much better when you're on the same page as your partner. The more you're able to speak up about your needs, the more fun it will be for both of you. Finding out what you like is important, and takes some experimentation. Sexual fantasies can be a big indicator of your wants and needs. Couples therapist Esther Perel says that fantasies are the ultimate secret code to what you want: they reveal your deepest wants and needs. She says how you were loved and how you were taught to connect both feed into how you are as a lover.

So it's your first time . . .

Having sex with a woman for the first time is nerve-wracking for anyone. Actually, it's more than that. We can downplay it and say it's not a big deal . . . but it is!! Especially if you feel like you have no idea what you're doing. Am I just going to fumble down there and hope for the best? Maybe you're excited and ready to hop into bed but it's OK if you're not. The great news is this sex is for you. So often sex in heterosexual relationships is for men. You have sex, they finish and that's it – they roll off and fall asleep and you're left staring at the ceiling as quick as they came. But sex with women is for both of you, and you can continue until you're both done. It can last as long as you both want it too. And the best part? Women know women's anatomy so naturally they know what feels good – not like a man digging around down there for gold, hoping to hit the jackpot.

Getting to know what feels good for you before having sex with your partner is great, because then you can tell them what you like and what doesn't work for you. Self-exploration isn't just an internal job! What turns us on as humans is constantly changing and depends on what we're going through in life. We have the power to turn ourselves on and off: it's not just down to another person.

And that's not just in sex. Being turned on is connecting to your life force, so things that excite you, like going to a concert or eating at your favourite restaurant, might turn you on (that's not to say you should whack out a vibrator in the middle of Sainsbury's, I might add). And the same goes for turning you off; someone being rude or having to hang up the washing might leave you feeling disconnected. For me? A big turn on is someone standing up for others; I don't necessarily want to rip that person's clothes off, but I have this feeling of aliveness that sparks inside me. When it comes to being turned on and off the power is always yours.

The same can be said for your libido. Very rarely do couples have the same libido and so there has to be some give and take. But one of the best things about lesbian sex? You never have to wait for a penis to recharge again. It's a marathon, and can last as long as you both want it to! But that's not to say you need to be having sex all the time – quality over quantity. It's better to be having really lovely sex, where you're both enjoying each other, than feeling like you're ticking a box with a weekly (or daily) meeting. Within lesbian sex there's a cliché called the 'lesbian death bed' – it basically refers to the idea that all lesbian relationships are doomed to end in no sex, women's libidos are generally lower than men's and other things take priority – even though lots of monogamous relationships end in the same way.

Energy, time and sex-drive all affect sex. My heterosexual friends literally have to schedule sex with each other because they're so comfortable in their relationship that they forget. And if they don't have sex they end up feeling like really great roommates rather than husband and wife.

Another cliché around gay sex is that there's a sub and a dom (a top and a bottom) – this is not always the case.

A 'top' in a lesbian relationship is generally the one who prefers giving rather than receiving sexual pleasure. Some tops will be happy to receive some of the time, but generally prefer giving. Some tops don't want to receive at all. People often assume that tops are the more masculine and more confident partners, but this is yet another stereotype. And a bottom is essentially the opposite of a top. 'Bottoms' tend to prefer to receive sexual pleasure than to give it. Most bottoms are happy to top occasionally, it's just their preference to receive.

It's also important to remember that just because you both have vaginas it doesn't mean you have the same taste when it comes to sex. Some prefer gentle, softer intimate encounters, others might like something a bit more thrilling. Check in with your partner continually. CONSENT doesn't go out the window just because there's no men involved, ladies. When approaching sex, especially for the first time, here are some questions to help you along:

- May I kiss you?
- Can we do [insert an activity you'd like to do here]?
- Can I take your clothes off?
- Would you like to have sex?

- I'd like to do or try [insert fun thing here]. What do you think about that?
- Is this comfortable for you?
- Are you enjoying yourself?
- Is there anything you'd like to try?
- Should I stop?
- Should I keep going?
- Are you comfortable with this?

Remember, consent can be withdrawn at ANY TIME so it's important to keep checking in with one another.

Trust me, there is no right or wrong way

Sex can still be sex with penetration using sex toys, but that's not the be-all and end-all for some people. Oral sex and scissoring are major players in the world of women loving women.

You might ask: what is scissoring? Scissoring might just be one of the most mythical sex acts of them all, one that is joked about, whispered about but very rarely explained to us properly. Scissoring is a way of having sex that's commonly associated with queer women, where partners rub their genitals together to achieve pleasure or orgasm.

Because scissoring figures so prominently in straight porn, some people believe things like 'real lesbians don't actually scissor'. On the other hand, there are some people who think that scissoring is the main or only way queer women have sex.

Overall scissoring is just you trying to find a comfortable position that creates pleasurable genital-to-genital contact, which is different for everyone. Finding what works with a given partner may also take time, as it's always about what works for both of you. You don't have to scissor for it to be sex, and you don't have to orgasm either. However, with lesbian sex, it's much more likely to happen!

Researchers at the University of Arkansas have discovered that although straight partners have sex more often, bisexual and lesbian women have more orgasms – by far. The study, conducted in 2018 with 2,300 respondents, found that women were 33 per cent more likely to orgasm when they were having sex with another woman. Sorry to all the guys out there, we just do it better! Or maybe we're just a bit more knowledgeable and generous with women's bodies? It makes sense, though: heterosexual sex has always prioritised a man cumming, and we know that penetrative sex is associated with the lowest orgasm frequency for women. If you want to make your partner orgasm, most people with vulvas need clitoral stimulation. Ask your partner how they like their clit to be touched or massaged, and remember that it might take some trial and error to get them there – and that's normal. Work on understanding how the clitoris works and getting familiar with the other parts of the vulva. The clitoris has one purpose, and one purpose only: to optimise sexual pleasure.

When women were asked in the same survey what makes sex pleasurable, two things came up most frequently: being present and being able to receive. Neither of these is about the physical things that take place during intercourse – they're both about connection. As women we're not great at receiving anything. When someone compliments what we're wearing, we either downplay it – 'Oh this old thing, I got it from a pigsty at Hackney Farm' – or we give it right back – 'So do you! You look amazing too!' Having trouble receiving in sex looks like when you get super-awkward or uncomfortable when sex becomes about you, and you'd rather focus on your partner. But our partners want us to have an enjoyable time too! It's OK, though: receiving is a skill you can practise (and not just in the bedroom). The next time someone gives you a compliment – do not compliment them back. See if you can sit there and hold it, without trying to hot potato it back to the other person. Say THANK YOU and nothing else.

If they give you flowers, it's up to you if you water them or not. If you practise receiving outside the bedroom, you'll feel more comfortable receiving in the bedroom.

Being present during sex can be hard, especially if you've had bad experiences in the past, but sometimes there are just other things on your mind, such as why is cheese now kept in lock boxes and the price of Lurpak. Your brain takes you elsewhere to avoid what's going on in the moment, but that's not much fun for your partner. Mindfulness is important during sex, as it means we're able to be present and in the moment with our partner.

So during the day, catch yourself when you are multitasking (stop brushing your teeth on the toilet, guys) and see if you can bring yourself back into the moment and concentrate on what you're doing and what's in front of you. It's OK if your brain takes you somewhere else during sex – it's just important that you acknowledge it with your partner.

Many of the women reading this will have experienced sexual trauma, be that sexual harassment, sexual assault or rape. According to a 2021 report published by the World Health Organization, one in four young women who have been in a relationship will have experienced violence from an intimate partner by the time they reach their mid-twenties. And as someone who has experienced sexual abuse at the hands of men, when it comes to sex, I'm scared. A part of my journey is learning how to explore that side of things safely and in a way where I feel like I'm in control. And do you know what? It is a big deal. So often we expect women to stay silent and just get over things, when actually these acts of abuse rock our core and can never be forgotten. Those memories often get reactivated when we're in a vulnerable position. We all come to sex with different histories and it's important to have those conversations with the person you want to have sex with. If you don't feel comfortable having those conversations, it could be a sign that you're not quite ready to take that next step. Most women are likely to have had some sort of bad experience sexually; and if not personally, they certainly will know someone who has. I don't have a single friend who hasn't got at least one story, so the chances are you could be on common ground, or at least won't have to explain in the same way you might if you were with a man. And if they have experienced it themselves they're more likely to understand and relate to how it's manifested in you.

While women don't feel as intimidating to me as men – that doesn't mean the feelings I have around sex don't cross over and bleed into current relationships. Staying in your body during sex is something many survivors have to learn. While it's safer to numb out, so you're not retriggered physically, it means you numb out from the positive sensations and feelings as well. Learning how to reconnect with your body is a cornerstone of healing and allows you to access something that is your birthright: pleasure.

We all deserve pleasure. We're biologically designed to experience it from birth. We know what feels good to us. It's our life force, our creativity, the soul of who we are.

For some of us, experiencing pleasure can bring feelings of guilt or shame, or we might feel selfish and undeserving. Being checked in or present is a learnt skill that takes practice and work, and it may seem strange at first to focus your attention on your experience. To practise being 'checked in', tune in to your own body, sensations, emotions and thoughts during sex. This will allow you to better experience the pleasure you can derive from sex. If you're like me and you're in your head 90 per cent of the time, it will take time to get the hang of this.

Here are three ways that can help us stay present while getting it on:

1   **Talk to your partner about what to look for when you're not present.** If you're having sex with your partner it may be useful to have this conversation before you get it on. Explain that sometimes you have a hard time being present during sex, and tell them if there are any signs they can look for. You can have a plan in place for what to do if that happens during sex so that both of you feel prepared and informed. Do you go non-verbal? Do you

have a hard time asking for what you need? Anything you can tell them will help both of you figure out how to proceed when this comes up so you can feel safe and connected to one another.

2 **Focus on your breath.** Breathing is a great way to come back to your body when you're elsewhere in thoughts. Concentrating on breathing in and out can help you return to the present and notice what's happening in your body and around you. If you notice that you feel most in your head and not in your body during sex, start taking some deep breaths in and out.

3 **Explore your senses.** Another way to practise embodiment during sex is to explore the information you're getting from your senses. It can be hard to take in all the sensations and information we get during sex, especially if we're used to tuning out or dissociating during sexual contact. It can be helpful to explore your senses one at a time, what are you feeling, what are you seeing, what are you hearing, to absorb what's going on. As you get more practice, it might become easier. Go sense by sense and see where you can bring awareness to what's going on in your body.

Sex should embrace three things: safety, connection and fun.

Girls just don't want to have STIs

Now we have our sexual knowledge down, I'm going to issue a mild warning: just because you're dating girls does not mean you're safe from STIs.

Those little infections get passed around in a multitude of ways. If one of you has an infection it can still be passed on through skin-to-skin touching, scissoring, oral sex or using the same hands on both of you. Fluids like discharge and saliva can carry STIs, so it's important we stay safe.

Because of the myth that lesbians can't get STIs, women dating women are much less likely to go for cervical cancer screenings because they think they're not at risk. Even if, like me, you all were marched out of your Year 9 history lesson and jabbed in the arm in the school hall with the HPV vaccine that meant you could barely lift your arm for forty-eight hours, girls fainting left right and centre, you still need to stay safe.

Most smear tests are so chill. Yeah, they're not the most comfortable thing in the world, but sing a bit of your favourite song and grit your teeth and it'll be over asap. My first one was done by a gynaecologist whose walls were adorned with photos of him and Rita Ora and who hurt me so badly I screamed and my best friend burst through the door to rescue me. I never went back. He still sends me Merry Christmas messages on WhatsApp. But having had many since then, I've barely felt them. And as for STI screenings, we have no excuses, girls – they're painless!

To be honest, women's healthcare is a mess, whatever your sexuality. We've only just discovered premenstrual dysphoric disorder (PMDD), that makes women depressed to the point of suicidal ideation each month. Navigating healthcare as a lesbian isn't necessarily a major issue, except that some doctors seem to not even consider that being a lesbian might be a real thing.

Case in point, this is a genuine conversation most gay girlies go through:

> 'Are you sexually active?'
>
> 'Yes.'
>
> 'Is there any chance you could be pregnant?'
>
> 'Nope!'
>
> Cue furrowed brow and scribbling.
>
> 'Are you sure? There's no way you could be?'
>
> 'Unless I'm the next chosen one for immaculate conception. Absolutely.'

I've heard stories of people being asked if their girlfriend was their sister, best friend and even mother. It's like they don't believe lesbians exist in the wild. The fact that doctors didn't even think to ask before taking a wild stab in the dark baffles me. What's next? Are they your dog walker? Your builder doing your extension? The lady on the phone renewing your car insurance? Let it be any of them, just not your GIRLFRIEND? 'We've done zero research on girls who date girls in the seven years it's taken us to train to be doctors.'

The healthcare experiences of lesbian and bisexual women are often overshadowed by research focused primarily on heterosexual females. There have been reports that have shown that lesbian and bisexual women seek healthcare less frequently, are less likely to go for mammograms and cervical screenings than our straight friends, says the Office of National Statistics (and it's not because lesbians are super-healthy as a result of our love of Whole Foods). This suggests that inaccessible healthcare, together with the worry of discrimination and homophobia in the healthcare system, contribute to decreased screening rates, putting LGBTQIA+ people at a greater risk of late-stage cancer diagnosis. So can doctors please get up to date and make us feel welcome and not like we've crashed a party we weren't invited to?

15

Why don't you just leave?

Dear Diary,

There's an insistent knocking on the door of our hotel room. I stumble towards it and open it a little, not wanting whoever's on the other side to see the mattress that's been flipped over and the chair strewn across the floor. I'm met by a large security guard and a man in a sharp navy suit who introduces himself as the hotel manager.

'We're just doing a welfare check. We've had phone calls from multiple rooms saying it sounds like a woman's in danger in this room. Are you OK, ma'am?'

They don't have to be Poirot to tell I'm the furthest thing from OK.

'Do you want us to take you to another room? It won't cost you anything.'

Every ounce of me wants to scream, 'Yes. Please get me out of here. Please take me away from this.' But my partner's standing behind me, and I know that if I do that it'll only make things worse in the long run.

My body's shaking as I whisper, 'I'm sorry for being a disturbance, we'll be quieter.'

'Are you sure?'

I can see the grave look on their faces, and one of them mouths 'Are you OK?'

They're desperately trying to get me to open up. They don't want to leave me in this room. Maybe they have daughters my age, or maybe they're just doing their jobs. But something is wrong. And they know.

'Yes, thank you. Thank you for your concern' and I mean it.

It's almost a relief. Seeing someone concerned about me, having hidden this part of my life for so long. Strangers heard what was going on and they wanted to help me . . . and when the calvary arrived I said no. Suddenly I am the women my mum used to tell me about from her days in the police. The women who, when the police were called couldn't speak up, even though it was evident what was happening.

I shut the door.

Jesus, how did I get here?

Rosie

When I started thinking about writing this book, I knew there was a chapter I desperately wanted to include, but knew that it might make people nervous. As a society we just can't keep pretending that this sort of thing doesn't happen. We need to look the beast right in the eye and not turn away. The more we sweep it under the rug, the more perpetrators get away with it and the more survivors feel they can't speak out. We carry the shame of what happened to us around in a rucksack every day – shame that is not ours to hold. And that shit gets heavy. This chapter may be hard to read, and I really appreciate you trying. If it's too much, please just skip ahead.

We have to acknowledge that abuse in relationships happens.

I was in a relationship that was at times abusive (although you were more likely to get me to vote for Donald Trump than admit it). I didn't think I was being abused – I thought I was being tolerant with an angry person. I had normalised watching household objects be punched, being screamed at and walking on eggshells, terrified of what was going to happen next. I used to think if I hadn't been shouted at, it had been a good day. The unpredictability left my nervous system in a state of constant freeze, unable to do anything except make sure my partner was OK at all times, judging his every move and sentence with as much skill as an Olympic gymnast commentator. When was he going to blow? How could I contain this situation? How could I navigate his moods?

Looking back, it was a textbook abusive relationship, laced with equal parts fear and my corrupted idea of love. It wasn't until a really bad day that I walked out and sat in the park in the rain. I watched as a group of Brownies played tag, remembering what it was to be eight years old. When I went home, I dropped to my knees and begged him to stop abusing me. He agreed, we made up . . . and then I waited for that promise to be broken. That night, lying in bed next to him, I finally confronted the truth: I needed to get out. And I had no idea how to do that.

Our relationship didn't start off with daily screaming rituals; it started with what I now know to be love bombing. Our first date lasted twenty-four hours, and we were together after a weekend. Two months later we had our own place. I was swept off my feet with attention, adoration, gifts and I LOVE YOUs. But even the most masterful manipulator can't hide forever – and at around the three-month mark, the first explosion happened. He was drunk, so I put it down to that, and he swore to never do it again. The explosions got more and more frequent – but the loving did too. Often people who are abusive are like pendulums, they can swing from one extreme to another – and fast.

He spotted what I needed, recognised my vulnerabilities and gave me everything I'd ever wanted, meaning my attachment to him was tied to my longing to be looked after. I wasn't aware of any of that at the time, of course. I was living blindly, trying to balance up the terror with the cuddles that would follow. All I knew was I couldn't tell anyone what was going on.

It wasn't until I got out of that relationship and slowly started opening up to people that I could no longer deny what had been happening. I wasn't educated on abusive behaviour, not in school, not by my parents, and I could justify everything I went through with a 'But he loves me'. There are many reasons why people are abused, and not a single one of them is their fault. For me, it all went back to childhood. If you grow up with an angry man in your house like I did, chances are that if you don't heal, you're going to repeat that cycle again. And that's what I did – but much, much worse this time.

The funny thing is that, deep down, I *did* know. I remember after one terrifying explosion a voice clear as anything saying, 'This is how it starts.' But I couldn't stop it. There was the time we were driving through a long tunnel and he started wrestling the steering wheel, making the car career across the road. We were going to hit the central reservation barrier. 'You're going to kill me,' I thought. But I couldn't stop it. Even when I got down on my knees and begged him to stop abusing me, the words finally pouring from my lips. But he didn't change. And still I stayed. As women, we've been taught to disown our 'No'. We've been conditioned to believe it has no value in the world. Our 'No' gets ground down, shaved off, belittled until it is a very tiny 'Yes'. We need to realise our 'No' is our best friend, our boundary and protector – and we must reclaim it.

In the quietest of moments, late at night, or on a walk with female friends I adored, I *did* know what was happening to me. I'd have this overwhelming urge to tell them. I was desperate for someone to see what was going on, but I couldn't admit it. If I admitted it to anyone, I'd have to leave. And being on my own seemed far scarier. My need for attachment was far greater than my need for safety: a dangerous state to be in. But, it turns out, my deepest fear happened to be the making of me. The relationship ended and I set out on a path of healing. I found solace in others who'd gone through similar things, went to therapy, read books that helped me heal and surrounded myself with as much support as possible. And I learnt being on your own is great. If I was a doctor I'd prescribe it. For at least two years in your twenties, YOU MUST BE SINGLE. It's full of self-discovery and exploration and is fucking great. I discovered neuroplasticity, that I could rewire my brain and live and think differently. Neuroplasticity is the brain's ability to change and adapt due to experience. Neuro refers to neurons, the nerve cells that are the building blocks of the brain and nervous system, plasticity refers to the brain's malleability or ability to change. Thus, neuroplasticity allows nerve cells to change or adjust and in doing so gives us opportunities to grow.

Learning to recognise the signs

What I've described happened to me in a heterosexual relationship, but sadly it's just as common in same-sex relationships.
More than one in ten LGBTQIA+ people (11 per cent) have
faced domestic abuse from a partner in the last year, according
to Stonewall.

Someone's gender does not determine whether they have
the capacity to be abusive, be that physically, emotionally or
sexually. It took years of work to undo what happened to me,
and I'd really like to stop the same thing happening to other
women.

When Casey met her girlfriend on a night out she was instantly
enamoured and things moved quickly. Within two months they
had moved in together. Casey's partner had a tendency to dig
at her under the guise of pretending to think things were 'cute'.
Casey's tummy, her print work as an artist, even a prize she was
awarded. Casey quickly clocked that her partner struggled to be
happy for her. In the bedroom, Casey was pressured into doing
things she wasn't comfortable with, but she complied because
she didn't want to exacerbate her partner's regular bad moods.

After a few intense months of dating, Casey went away for
a week for work. On coming back her partner seemed distant.
After checking her partner's tags on Instagram and seeing her
cuddled up with another woman at a party, she realised her
partner had cheated on her. When she confronted her about
it, her partner made out that Casey was the problem in the
relationship, being too clingy and pushing her away, putting
too much pressure on her. Casey's partner became critical of
her, regularly berating her for forgetting household tasks, or for

going out with friends. Her moods became more erratic and her anger manifested in books and plates being thrown around their apartment. The more Casey tried to pull away, the more fury was directed at her. Her partner even threatened to harm herself should Casey leave. It wasn't until Casey was out for a meal with a friend and her partner called her twenty-seven times that her friend sounded the alarm bell; and at long last Casey confided how she'd been living. Her friend made plans for Casey to stay with her and her partner until she could safely extricate herself from the relationship.

Only when Casey was fully out of the relationship did she realise just how bad it had been. When you're so close to something, you can't always see what's right in front of your face. When you think you love someone, you'll excuse anything – and everything.

So firstly, let's get clear on the basics of abuse, that lesson that was conveniently left off the school timetable. When I was first taught about this, the cogs turned and the jigsaw pieces slotted into place; suddenly what had been happening made sense. I felt ashamed for not knowing these things before, but when no one's taught you it, it's no different from expecting you to know how to speak Mandarin on the fly.

Physical abuse

This is one of the first forms of domestic abuse that people recognise because it's the most visible. We've often seen TV series and films depict women with black eyes and bruised faces, or flinching away from their partners. Physical abuse is a common way for a perpetrator to gain control: hitting, slapping, spitting, choking, hair pulling or using an object to attack you. It can also include punching walls and breaking objects. I spent a lot of money replastering my walls after having someone's knuckles smash through them – at the time I didn't realise that physical abuse didn't just mean physically hurting you, but also includes physically threatening behaviour. And FYI it is illegal. All of this is.

Psychological and emotional abuse

This can be difficult to describe or identify if you live with it day to day because it becomes normalised. It's when a perpetrator uses words and non-physical actions to manipulate, hurt, scare or upset you. Some examples of this abuse are screaming and shouting at you, making threats, mocking you and making degrading comments. The abuser will say that the abuse is your fault, tell you they're sorry and that their behaviour doesn't count as abuse. I once convinced myself that getting six phone calls a day, where I was screamed at, was as normal as a trip to the supermarket. Your brain is hardwired for survival, and not picking up those calls would have put me in greater danger in the long run. As a result I still struggle to take phone calls (but also because – guys, it's 2025 – just WhatsApp me).

Sexual abuse and violence

This can also take place within relationships. If you give in to something because you are afraid or you have been pressured into it, it is not consent. Rape or sexual assault are both examples of sexual abuse, as is any sexual act you did not consent to. It can include forced kissing, touching or penetration, and having sex with you when you are unable to consent, for example if you are under the influence of drugs or alcohol. Using force, threats, guilt, manipulation or intimidation to make you perform sexual acts is also abuse. Sometimes you can consent to have sex, but what actually follows is not what you agreed. You have every right to change your mind and withdraw your consent. Someone asking you over and over again, and you eventually relenting to get them to stop, is not OK either.

Coercive control

This is controlling behaviour designed to make a person dependent on the perpetrator by isolating them from support, exploiting them, depriving them of independence and regulating their everyday behaviour. Coercive control creates invisible chains and a sense of fear that pervades all elements of a victim's life. It works to limit their human rights by depriving them of their liberty and reducing their ability for action. Experts such as American sociologist Evan Stark liken coercive control to being taken hostage. As he says in his book *Coercive Control*: 'The victim becomes captive in an unreal world created by the abuser, entrapped in a world of confusion, contradiction and fear.'

Financial abuse is part of coercive control, and involves a pattern of controlling, threatening and degrading behaviours relating to money and finances. The perpetrator uses money to control their partner's freedom. This can include using their credit or debit cards without permission or building up debts in their partner's name. Economic abuse is a broader term, as it also includes restricting access to essential resources and services, such as food, clothing or transport, and refusing to allow someone to improve their economic status through employment, education or training.

Gaslighting

If you live online, you'll have heard the term gaslighting used in TikToks and Insta reels from self-help accounts. Gaslighting makes you doubt your own sanity. A perpetrator may gaslight you into thinking that you are misremembering or misinterpreting things, later making you believe that their version of events is the truth. This behaviour is used to manipulate a person.

It's important to remember that perpetrators will justify their actions so that they can place blame on survivors and remove any responsibility from themselves.

So how can abuse play out in same-sex relationships? An abuser can use the fact that their victim is LGBTQIA+. These can include:

- Threats to 'out', i.e. to disclose someone's sexual orientation or gender identity without their consent, for example to their employer, family or community.

- Criticising someone for not being a 'real lesbian or bisexual woman', for example if they have only recently come out or previously been in a heterosexual relationship.

- Playing on fears that no one will help because someone 'deserves' the abuse.

- Playing on the belief that agencies (like the police) are prejudiced against the LGBTQIA+ community.

There are also a number of myths about domestic abuse that can prevent people from getting help. Sometimes an abuser will use these myths to try and stop someone reporting their experiences (e.g. to the police), thereby giving the abuser free rein to do whatever they like.

If you're new to the LGBTQIA+ community an abusive partner may explain their bad behaviour by saying something like, 'This is how it is in a lesbian or bisexual woman's relationship.' Other times, they may say that abuse only happens in heterosexual relationships and can't happen between two women.

It's amazing what the brain will do to gaslight you into thinking everything is OK and normal. Your brain will choose familiarity over new, scary experiences. This is that happened to me: the idea of leaving that relationship, giving up my life as I knew it, was too overwhelming, so my brain made what was going on in the relationship OK. I came up with a million excuses for their behaviour. I justified what was happening to me, and I believed I deserved it.

'Why don't you just leave?'

A question that's on the lips of even the most well-intentioned person is: 'Why don't you just leave?' My answer is: 'How do you escape a system that's designed to keep you trapped?' A maze of attachments that can't just be broken by packing a suitcase and calling an Uber. So many people want life to be that simple. Many cannot understand why you would allow yourself to be treated in such a way. People seem to be more concerned about why someone stays in abusive relationships than why abusers abuse. Victim blaming is still alive and well. There will always be someone who will find a way to turn it back on you and make it your fault. It's not.

And the people who are baffled by it? They need to go and educate themselves. Maybe they were lucky and had someone teach them what is OK and what's not! But the truth is that until you're in that situation it's impossible to know how you'd react. People often say 'trust your gut instinct' – I was in my twenties, and I hadn't yet developed one. And people don't understand it: it's not just the abuse, it's the people who turn a blind eye, who act like it never happened, who can't discuss your life with you. It's the people who expect you to have moved on, to get over it. It's the lack of consequences, the lack of resources, it's the surviving after the surviving.

What people don't understand is that the decision to stay is not always a choice. Often the attachment is so strong to your abuser, because of their clever manipulation, that losing them feels unsurvivable. I was told regularly often in a jovial way, 'You wouldn't survive without me. You can't do anything on your own.' And I learnt to believe that. It's no wonder I was terrified to face the world alone. I genuinely thought I was incapable of survival without that relationship. People seemed to think that leaving was as easy a decision as cancelling a Deliveroo order. Delete the katsu curry, Rosie, AND WALK AWAY. Nope. Often you become so enmeshed with your partner, it feels impossible to extricate yourself.

'Why didn't you go to the police?' Is another one. Firstly, I didn't know any of this was illegal – and, babe, have you seen how the police support women? I have more chance of winning the lottery than the police coming through for me with a charge. It's so hard wanting justice for yourself but also having to weigh up the pain and trauma of reliving your experience with such a small hope of any result I had to ask myself, was it worth it?

In the end I chose to heal. Which happened in the tiniest of baby steps, one day at a time. I had to come to terms with what had happened, I had to unpick all the unhealthy messaging I had internalised, and I had to feel all the emotions I had put a lid on for a number of years. The pain, the fear, the grief, the anger. The analogy about running water is true. When you first turn on a rusty old tap it's hard, it's stiff, it's a struggle. The water is brown and murky, but slowly as you let it run, it becomes less cloudy until finally it runs clear. Transitioning to a life of safety, of calm, at first felt strange, I was so used to living off adrenaline I felt . . . bored. But then the boredom made way for being grounded, for navigating the world from a place of being centred and in tune with who I was despite it all, and what I wanted.

You deserve to live a life where you feel happy and safe. That is your birthright. Love is not fear. Love is secure. Love is authenticity. And love is sometimes . . . uneventful. Love is not what we see in the movies. Love is in the everyday.

How to seek help

So what do you do if you recognise that you're in an abusive relationship? It's so easy for me to write this with hindsight, knowing how difficult it is at the time. Even if I had read this book when in that relationship, I'd probably still have felt that it was impossible to leave.

Reach out to one person you trust. A friend, a family member or someone you feel a connection with. The fear you have of speaking out will be met by compassion and a desire to help you through the situation. Trying to leave on your own, while totally possible, is hard, and having someone alongside you is only going to help you. Make a plan of how to get safe – is there somewhere you can stay? Is it possible for you to pack your bags and leave? If not, is there a women's shelter you can reach out to? Every relationship and every situation is unique, as is every break-up, so it's important to create a plan to end the relationship safely. Once you have the physical plans in place you can tackle the incredibly painful bit.

Once you've left, you have to block your abuser. There is no other way. If they have the ability to contact you, they will find a way to reach you and worm their way back in. I had to change my email address three times during our separation because there was always something he needed to talk to me about. And when I wouldn't talk to him, that would often lead to threats of self-harm. This is such a common tool of manipulators – they will threaten they're going to self-harm or even kill themselves if you don't get back with them. I remember the moment when I genuinely believe my life was saved. Me and my ex had split up but he was finding excuses to contact me. I was still living in the same house, and after I told this person that he'd turned up unexpectedly one day she looked me straight in the eye and spoke in a tone I'd never heard before. Such gravity and control. 'Activate the break clause, Rosie.' I realise this sentence sounds like something from a *Star Wars* scene when they're trying to control the spaceship – but those five words saved my life. It meant all ties were cut from him. It meant I had a chance of freedom, of space in which to heal. Which is messy and non-linear and goddamn hard. The truth is, it's going to hurt. It hurts and hurts and hurts until slowly one day at a time, it hurts less. It's not about feeling better, it's about allowing the feelings to be there. To sit with the pain until it moves through you. It takes time to process what has happened and the effect it may have had on your mind, body and life. Sometimes you need distance to see the truth. Even now, I can still get triggered by things that bring me back to that place but I know if I allow the feeling to be present, it's much more likely I can move through it and continue with my day.

Reconnecting with loved ones, friends and people in your community, especially if you've been isolated from them during your relationship can also be so helpful as you heal. Many believe there's no help available for abusive relationships within the LGBTQIA+ community, which is simply not true. My gay superhero movie will of course include Rebel Wilson bursting into houses and throwing abusers out of windows, but until then there are places to reach out to if you do find yourself in this situation.

GALOP

Galop's helpline is run by LGBT+ people for LGBT+ people who have or are experiencing domestic abuse. It's also for people supporting a survivor of domestic abuse: friends, families and those working with a survivor. It's free and accessible through phone, Webchat and Chatbot.

Switchboard LGBT+ Helpline

This provides a safe space for anyone to discuss anything, including sexuality, gender identity, sexual health and emotional well-being. They support people to explore the right options for themselves and aspire to a society where all LGBT+ people are informed and empowered.

Victim Support

This is a service I've used myself. After reaching out to them and having an initial phone call where we talked through what had happened, they assigned me a case worker. I remember feeling so embarrassed relaying everything to them: I felt like such a fool. How could I have let that happen to me? Every time my ex contacted me I would reach out to my case worker and she would log it. That way everything was documented and prepared should the police need it for evidence. They also sent me self-aid kits for my home. At Victim Support I was met with nothing but such kindness and understanding.

16

How to heal from heartbreak

Dear Diary,

I cried on the floor of Sainsbury's takeaway aisle.

I watched the films you hated.

Listened to the artist you used to roll your eyes at.

Tried drinking red wine.

Took up vaping.

Hated red wine.

Went for a run.

Forgot I have the stamina of a teenage boy experiencing his first time.

Dyed the ends of my hair pink.

Spilt red wine on the carpet.

Stopped running.

Can't open the fridge because we used to dance in the kitchen.

Cut up your shirts.

Chopped my hair into a bob.

Buried my face in the strips of your shirt.

Took a pottery class then smashed the bowl against a wall.

Re-read our messages.

Spilt dinner down my pyjamas and didn't change them.

Told everyone I'm over you.

Re-read our messages again.

Moved my sofa to the living room and build a fort.

Screamed 'We Are Never Ever Getting Back Together' at the top of my lungs.

Cried on the bathroom mat to Adele.

Ordered the same Deliveroo for a month.

Thought about getting hit by a car to get your attention.

Went to yoga.

Blocked your number.

Stalked your Instagram on my friends' phones.

Talked about you so much my friends vetoed the topic.

Learnt to cook my favourite meal.

Learnt to live without you.

Learnt how to find me.

Love,

Rosie x

It's a truth universally acknowledged that unless you're dead inside, most break-ups SUCK. Even with the latest Taylor Swift album to scream along to, you're still left trying to process and figure out what life now looks like without that one person. By all accounts, lesbian break-ups can feel like you just got locked out of your house except the keys are now in the Indian Ocean and you're going to have to figure out how to get there, scuba dive *and* not get eaten by a great white shark – just to get home and feel normal again. There are meme accounts entirely dedicated to lesbian break-ups. They can be intense. Inhale the self-help books (lol, hello) and the podcasts, and sit with your friends who, between sips of red wine, will tell you they never liked them anyway and you can do way better.

Sometimes it feels like there aren't the words to articulate how heavy a broken heart can feel. You're grieving for someone who's still alive, yet you're expected to carry on as usual. There's no funeral. No two weeks off and often no closure. Maybe we should start holding funerals for our exes? Rather than cremating them we just burn their stuff? What if we took heartbreak more seriously? Above all, what would happen if we looked at what we've gained from a relationship, however long it lasted, as well as what we've lost?

Especially in your first lesbian relationship. You've made what might have felt like the impossible, possible. Very often your first relationship is tied into the joy and elation of you coming out, of being who you truly are. The end of that can feel like the party's ended and you're left alone to cry on the dance floor. Coming out may have been something you dreamed about for years and so the end of that first relationship is going to feel crushing. And when a relationship ends we often have the fear that we're never going to find another person again. 'PLENTY MORE FISH IN THE SEA.' Yes, but I want THAT very specific, ridiculous piece of salmon, please.

As we touched on briefly earlier, a common thing amongst lesbian relationships is enmeshment, which is not the healthiest thing in the world. Someone in an enmeshed relationship is overly connected to the other person's needs and so loses touch with their own needs, goals, desires and feelings. If you are enmeshed, the separation is like trying to detach a whole part of you from your very core. You have the same friends. You do the same activities. You're close with their parents. If your family didn't respond well to you coming out, you may have become super-close with theirs. There's a sticky lesbian glue effect: as women, we bond so deeply at an alarming speed, so we end up committing to each other before we're actually ready to. And when you realise you're perhaps not as compatible as you first thought, untangling yourself from the other is like peeling a human body off one of those giant Velcro walls.

It may be that queer women don't have a strong network of other queer women who they can talk to, while men or women in heterosexual relationships tend to have a bigger pool of literature, information and media to call upon, so queer women are left in the heartbreak alone. The world you'd craved for so long, now gone. The good news is that in lesbian relationships it's very common you'll end up being friends. My friend has many of her exes at her birthday parties and it's just something that's accepted. Queer friendships and our community are so vital to our lives and survival (safety in numbers) that after processing the pain, you often find a way through to stay friends with your exes (with some healthy boundaries in place, I might add). If you find yourself in a period of isolation QueerTok has become its own universe of queer community and acceptance. Queer spaces can be physical – and that's great – but people might live at home, or with their parents, or in a small place where there is no one to talk to. The internet can be a space to process all of it.

A relationship that's ended can either be a waste of time or something you learnt from. You get to decide; you get to give it meaning. You can be heartbroken and pissed off, but you can turn it on its head to focus on what the relationship has taught you and where you're going next. 'I'll never be the same again,' you cry into your fourth bowl of Coco Pops – and it's true. You won't be. You'll be wiser. You'll have had an experience that will set you up to make other experiences less painful and more manageable. Most of us are heartbroken more than once in our lives, and a well-trodden map is useful to have within our grasp.

Breaking up without breaking apart

Some break-ups are easier and for the best for everyone; others make you want to scream into a void for weeks on end. Either way, it's not a pleasant experience. But what should you do afterwards? When you can't stop thinking about the person who broke your heart, how do you actually move on?

As a very wise woman once told me (and then told me again and again because I wasn't listening) *The worst thing that will ever happen to you is that you will have a feeling.* We have to feel our feelings. If we don't, they get buried and burst out or spill over in situations where we might not want them to. Lots of us are scared of our feelings. We've categorised them into good and bad: 'happy' = good; 'sad and crying' = bad. But feelings have no morality. They're simply energy that needs to be released and a cycle completed. We often feel better after a massive cry because we've released something that was trapped. With feelings, the only way out is *through*. Like *We're Going on a Bear Hunt*, 'We can't go over it, we can't go under it, we have to go through it' – except we're not meeting a bear at the end of it. We're meeting our healed self.

If you're worried about feeling sad all day, give yourself a set amount of time where you allow yourself to sit with the sadness. For fifteen minutes, put on a sad song and really express what your body needs to. If you're angry, whack your sofa or bed with a pillow. Heck, even screaming into a pillow is an excellent way of releasing pent-up emotions. But what's important is that you get them out safely and don't let them fester.

What can you do when you find yourself in a woman-loving-woman (or maybe in this case woman-hating-woman) break-up?

- **Talk about it.** You don't have to go through this alone. Your friends are your best support system, so rant and rave to them. If you have a community of LGBTQIA+ pals, turn to them and ask how they got through similar situations.

- **Don't expect too much of yourself too soon.** It can take time to process and heal. If it's a relationship that's run into years, it may take anything up to that amount of time to fully exit your system.

- **Reflect.** If on reflection it wasn't a great relationship for you, what do you need to do so that you don't take it forward into the next relationship and create a cycle?

- **Understand that your break-up could be preparing you for something better.** The universe knows what it's doing (if you're into that kind of thing) and there might be someone else better suited to you.

- **Set boundaries with your ex.** I know you really want to text them or reply to that funny meme they posted on

their Instagram. Don't do it. Enforce your boundaries
– I like to give myself sixty days of no contact. You
might want to see how you feel after a month at first;
even if you do still want to reach out you'll be in a
different place mentally and maybe physically (trip to
Cancun anyone?) by then.

- **Do not return to the person who hurt you.** The person
  who hurt you will not heal you.

- **Just get the haircut.** We both know you're going to do it.

One of the many things they don't teach us in schools is how to
end a relationship. Sure, we might be excellent at being broken
up with, but how do we become the breakee? This often leads
to people staying in a relationship because they feel obligated.

So how do we break up with people in a way that's healthy
for both parties? It might not go the way you planned, but
sometimes knowing you behaved in a decent way gives you
the peace you might not otherwise have. We all want to end
with some dramatic line that sounds like it's from a blockbuster
movie, but a) thinking of one in the moment is really hard and
b) the conversations we rehearse in our heads never do go as
planned. Sure, sometimes you do have to throw their clothes
out on to the street when you find out they've been cheating on
you for three years. But for your average relationship that's run
its course, here are some things to consider when you're the one
who's ending it.

- We're all too mature (are we?) to end things over
  text or a phone call. I broke up with someone over

the phone once, and it was a shitty thing to do. No
matter how hard the conversation is going to be,
do it face to face in a neutral space. A space from
where you can both leave afterwards. My friend's
partner ended things after five years in her favourite
restaurant across the street from her house. I'm all for
exposure therapy, but that seems unnecessarily cruel.
He also quoted the bridge from Taylor's 'Champagne
Problems' about the bride being 'fucked in the head'.
BRUTAL.

- If the relationship has just fizzled out and you want
  to move on, be clear about your intentions and
  reasons. This doesn't apply if there are extenuating
  circumstances like affairs or abuse, but if you've fallen
  out of love with someone, it's good to have an honest
  conversation about that. This is not a time to throw in
  Taylor's, 'There will be no explanation there will just be
  reputation.'

- Say what you need to say, be honest, be respectful
  and listen to what the other person wants you to hear.
  You're not responsible for their emotions or reactions,
  but your behaviour has an impact and it's good to be
  aware of that.

- For the love of God, don't ghost someone you're
  in a relationship with, even if it was a short one.
  Even me, chief ghoster of my friends (I have the
  attachment style of a cat – I disappear for a month
  and then demand love and food). We have to learn to
  communicate when things aren't working for us, so we

don't go around wounding one another. How would you feel if someone just ghosted you? Let's remember empathy here.

● Try to avoid break-up sex. Elongated arguments that turn into sex on the sofa make things confusing in the long run. The hormones released during sex can temporarily make you feel differently about your ex and then you're in a sticky situation when you wake up the next day and remember the reasons why you actually don't want to be in a relationship with them.

● Don't play games or string them along with the chance you may get back together. This isn't a Netflix romcom of will they, won't they? Make sure you're clear about your decision.

● Having said be honest, you can be economical with the truth. Not EVERYTHING has to be said. We can't all just go around saying exactly what we feel at all times in some veiled attempt at 'being authentic' – so often people hide under a veil of speaking their truth – but not everything that's in your head needs to come out of your mouth. I'm not suggesting we should all walk on eggshells and be afraid to speak up, but words can hurt people and stay with them for a very long time. You should try to be fair, kind, honest and clear.

If you're on the receiving end of any of the above, it's still impossibly hard. When you've suffered a kitchen floor reset (when you're hysterically crying on your kitchen floor at 2 a.m. eating hummus with a fork), it can feel like it's impossible to keep going. It's like a tsunami of pain and you are a very inexperi-enced surfer, and when you think you might be over it you get eaten by a great white shark of memories. After one of my break-ups, I put together a pretty solid list of reasons to stay alive that in the midst of the snot, messy buns and five-day-old pyjamas, which might just lift you a little. After all, we need hope. So, REASONS TO KEEP GOING WITHOUT THEM:

- The new series of *The Traitors* (other TV series are available).
- There's a dog in your future you haven't met yet.
- Customer service so awful it makes you laugh.
- Claudia Winkleman's fringe.
- Getting to rearrange your apartment (or move!) and create a space that's just for you.
- Cheese! Have you had melted cheese? Pizza? There is so much cheese to be eaten and we must not take this for granted.
- Sunshine. Are you just sad, or is it just raining?
- Really good bread and butter.
- Asking for help and getting the help you need. Asking for help is giving people the chance to love you. Let them.
- The kind of hugs that heal your body, when you can feel the weight being lifted off your shoulders.
- Those one-off nights out that were just meant to be an early dinner but turn into you wearing a cowboy hat at 1 a.m. and being sung at by the rest of the bar.

- Crisp, sunny mornings.
- New babies who belong to people you love, who will grow up to love you.
- Long talks with old friends who put the world to rights with you. Long talks with new friends who make you feel seen and alive.
- Clean bed sheets (worth the nightmare of getting stuck inside the duvet cover and running into a wall in the process).

Because one day, all the days will have added up, and you realise that you're in a totally different place with little idea of how you got there – but suddenly everything is different and you're proud of yourself.

Healing from a relationship is weird, because sometimes you'll be sobbing violently on the bathmat over your ex from a year ago and then you'll just get up and go to the shops and buy dinner and take your little bit of sadness around with you until it feels less heavy. That's the thing about it: it makes itself known in the little moments. The faint breaths of relief, when you suddenly realise your chest isn't as tight any more. A night out with friends where you don't think about them. When you don't fear someone talking to you. The first morning where you wake up and see flowers on your windowsill and you don't feel scared, because you remember that flowers always turn towards the light. The first day you don't cry and you don't want to. You're learning how to live again having survived the storm – that's a universal experience for us all.

You might not be the same person you were, but you can still be fully whole.

And remember, not all exes are bad. I mean, look at you – you're someone's ex and you're pretty damn great.

17

Lesbi long term

Dear Diary,

I've ventured out on a train, a plane and a taxi, and now I'm staying in a tiny inn that looks like something out of a horror film – somewhere in Scotland – for my best friend's wedding. The whole thing's cost me about £800 (OK, I didn't need to buy a new dress) and I'm filled with excitement and butterflies for the day that lies ahead. The wedding has taken up most of my friend's year. She has planned everything down to a T, the prices for flowers making me wince – I want the day to be perfect for her. She walks down the aisle looking like a supermodel, we all cry at the vows. We eat lovely food, laugh at pitch-perfect speeches and then dance the night away to The Spice Girls. I wander back to the inn with a macaroni and cheese pie in one hand, my heels in another. It was completely delightful. The two of them make me believe in love. But . . .

    I just don't quite get it.
    Am I a commitment-phobe?

Love,
Rosie x

OK, I'm the first one to admit . . . I don't really understand marriage. How can you be sure that you're not going to say yes to someone and then, a year later, the love of your life walks by . . . and suddenly you're going to have to break someone's heart to get what you want? As a people pleaser this is my stuff of nightmares. There are around eight billion people on the planet – but I can't meet them all and then choose? I like to know all my options before making a life-changing decision. And even then I'm the most indecisive person ever, so will never actually make a choice. The pressure to pick a partner and stay with them for life seems daunting. I can barely choose a new pair of jeans without a breakdown, and I can at least take them back to the shop if I change my mind. But many people are not commitment-phobes like me and are after the big white wedding spectacular or are open to long-term commitment without marriage.

Weddings do puzzle me . . . you're paying £60,000 for a dinner and a DJ? I got that for £3.50 at my Year 3 disco with some Space Raiders thrown in. And you're playing the same songs, guys – I've been to three weddings this year and 'Valerie' was played at all of them! My friend went to thirty-one weddings in one year. She spent more time travelling to the weddings than actually being there!

I hate to be the bearer of bad news, but lesbian marriages have a divorce rate twice higher than men in same-sex relationships. A report published by the Office of National Statistics revealed that 67.2 percent of couples that petitioned for divorce in 2021 were female. I see this is as a positive, in a way. If something's not working for us, we feel confident enough to walk away.

Being in love and going through the whole wedding scenario gets expensive and demanding. Think about it: on average you speak to your guests for three minutes per person. I did peak at my friend's wedding who sent us on safari between the wedding and dinner, so instead of standing around making chitchat with Uncle Brian, we got loaded into trucks and went off to see lions and giraffes! Maybe I only like weddings with themes? *Don't Tell the Bride* style? Maybe I struggle to believe in love lasting forever when we're shown so many examples of how it doesn't. We're in a cozzie living crisis – is getting married financially viable? And just because you're married, it doesn't mean you need to stop working on your relationship. Your marriage will constantly evolve and change, and will sometimes be tested. It's something that needs to be grown and cherished. The good news is that more couples than ever are turning to couples' therapy and realising that strong relationships take work.

Amelia and Kye found themselves in couples' therapy after they 'lost the plot' six years into their marriage, soon after having a baby daughter. They like this phrase after hearing a divorce lawyer use it – couples who end up in his office have often 'lost the plot' of their relationship, like a book plot that wanders away and never gets back on track. Amelia and Kye went to couples' therapy for six months to get to the root of their issues, a mixture of confused priorities and fighting over the need to always be in the right. They both agree they could have just walked away – that would have been easier – but realising how much their relationship had changed after the birth of their daughter meant they needed to revisit who they both were at this stage of life and find out whether they could work through their issues together. They learnt that making rash decisions in the first few years of their child's life was not a wise idea; they were both so sleep-deprived they kept missing each other entirely. They say their relationship is now stronger than ever, having negotiated this rough patch, and that they now communicate in a way that works for their whole family.

Are you ready for 'I do'?

So if you kick me, old misery guts, aside, what do you do when you think you've found THE ONE? The love of your life, the Jay-Z to your Beyoncé, through thick or thin . . . What do we do? Do we go for a marriage v. civil partnership v. why are we bothering with this archaic institution? Does marriage equal equality, or are we all in it for the tax break? Can't be marrying money (like every middle-aged woman advised when we were growing up) when our partners are more often than not stuck under the same glass ceiling as we are . . . puts a different slant on the gender pay gap, doesn't it?

Our first option is the civil partnership. This act allowed same-sex couples to obtain legal recognition of their relationship (thanks government for noticing we are real and not in fact aliens). It blows my mind that this happened only twenty years ago. However, *marriage* between same-sex couples only became legal in 2013. Since the legal consequences of marriage or civil partnership are pretty much the same, it really comes down to personal choice. Should the relationship go tits up (no pun intended), a marriage ends in divorce, whereas a civil partnership is dissolved. In both cases, it's done through the courts. What's nice is that it finally feels on a par with heterosexual couples.

Religion and homophobia create one of the biggest barriers to the LGBTQIA+ community when it comes to weddings. We're banned from some churches in case we go up in flames when we walk down the aisle and it's Notre-Dame all over again. When people say they oppose marriage in same-sex couples what they're essentially saying is: 'I am fine with denying other people equal rights, on account of tradition, even though their exercise of equal rights does not deprive me of anything.' When people reference [insert holy text] and say it's wrong to be gay, I'm like . . . can you show me the small print, please?

What about the other things that the Scriptures mention are forbidden but which people ignore? Why is the focus on singling out LGBTQIA+ identities for criticism? We're not nailing people to crosses for stealing loaves of bread any more – please, come get with the times. And if they hold the belief that God created everything, then God created us too (a hell of a lot of us, actually). When it comes to marriage it's understandable that many of us don't desire to get married as it's tying ourselves to an institution that doesn't respect who we are.

As my purple-haired, iconic friend Ellen Jones writes in her book *Outrage*, there was significant contention over whether same-sex marriage should be allowed in the UK, or whether civil partnerships were enough. While there are innumerable issues with the historic institution of marriage and many still choose to have civil partnerships in light of this, the very existence of civil partnerships provided a convenient way for those who didn't really support LGBTQIA+ people to claim they believed in their right to marry. Even UKIP, one of the UK's further right political parties at that time, ostensibly supported LGBTQIA+ people's right to marry, but claimed that no action was needed because it essentially already existed in the form of civil partnerships. A right which they claimed to respect.

If you choose to get married, a question I've asked myself over and over again is: what do you do with your last names, when two women get married to each other? I was always pretty pissed that every surname originates from a man. Your surname is your dad's, and his was his dad's and then when heterosexual couples marry, you get your husband's – and even if you choose to keep your surname, you're still keeping your dad's! At no point did women get a surname that they got to choose. I'd like to put an end to that and create a whole new surname for me and my children. Something sexy and aloof like Delacroix . . . And being gay might be an excellent reason to do that.

When I speak to Maddy and Emily, now happily married for three years, they originally didn't agree on marriage. Maddy had dreamed of her wedding day since she was a little girl; she has photos of her dressed up in her mother's wedding dress, Emily had always thought it wasn't for her and was pretty set on her freedom. When Emily realised how important it was to Maddy, they had many discussions (and a few arguments) about what was right for them. What settled it in the end was the security that marriage would provide for them and their future children, and them both promising to divorce amicably should the need ever arise. In the end they had a civil ceremony at a court house in their city, followed by what sounded like a magical woodland ceremony with their friends and family. They took each other's names, creating a double-barrelled surname. They say married life feels no different from before – it was never about the truth of their love – but that there's a foundation now from which their relationship can grow.

18

The kids are alright

Dear Diary,

One of the most painful states of being is imagining the future you know you're never going to have. I've known I've wanted a baby since I unwrapped a BABY born doll on my third Christmas morning and, despite scribbling on its face in black biro, I was obsessed. It went everywhere with me: to nursery, to bed, in the bath. I was better at feeding that BABY born than I was at feeding myself (I'd learnt how to be a selfless mother at three, how clever). I soon learnt that Santa wasn't real, too. One Christmas Eve I laid my bassinet next to my bed and asked Santa to bring me a real baby to look after. Imagine my devastation when I was not woken by tiny gurgles and minute fingernails but instead an empty basket and stocking filled with chocolate.

I felt my parents' betrayal all day. How could they get away with this lie? They knew how much I wanted a baby sibling. I'd balanced my little body over the pram of my best friend's newborn sister so often that the teachers assumed it was my sibling. By the end of every summer holiday I'd be running my own kids' club, a trail of tiny sandals flip-flopping after me. Even now I ask people if I can steal their babies. Just last week, at my friend's birthday, she told her friend to hold on to his five-week-old in case I lobbed her in my handbag and ran off. Is it really kidnapping if I'm a lovely person and take really good care of her?

My dream of living a Gilmore Girls *mother–daughter relationship like Lorelai and Rory seems a distant possibility. I want to drink pumpkin spice lattes and gossip and go shopping and have a teenage girl slam a door in my face . . . before the inevitable cuddling up on the sofa in our matching pyjamas. Is that so much to ask? Why do I have to lose out on something just because I'm gay? And not only that, something I've dreamed of my entire life?*

The thing that caused me the most pain in all of this claiming my sexuality affair was the realisation I was never going to have a baby by accident. There would be no midnight fumbles and 'I think I might be pregnant' panic/excitement moments. No rushing to the shops still feeling fifteen as I pay for a pregnancy test (even now, when my friends have babies, I think it must be impossible as we are still only teenagers, and we are in fact teen mums). There would be no lovely surprises and no decisions to make. And I felt robbed. Why can't I have a child as easily as my heterosexual counterparts?

I realised that if I wanted a baby biologically, I was probably going to have to pay for one with cold hard cash . . . Although recently the NHS has granted LGBTQIA+ prospective parents the same rights as heterosexual couples, allowing them up to three cycles of IVF for free. I can't help but think it would be much easier if they sold them on Amazon, but instead I was going to have to be harvested like a field, my eggs kept on ice and then re-implanted into me. I think about it most days, about what that journey will be like, as I've heard from so many that it's not a walk in the park. It feels unfair. Sure, I could buy sperm on the internet from a stranger and keep my legs up for half an hour, but that comes with risks I'm not totally down with, like my baby loving football, and I just can't do that to myself.

I'm disappointed women haven't evolved into being able to reproduce by themselves like worms. Yes, that's correct. Worms don't have sex. I would happily be a worm if I could make a child myself or grow back a new leg if someone pulled me in two. But since I am in fact a human, I have four options: adoption; IVF; surrogacy; stealing a baby from Sainsbury's. Only one comes with potential jail time, but to be honest it seems the easiest to pull off.

Love,

Rosie x

No, this bit is not an ode to one of the only films I know showing a lesbian couple parenting. This is all about babies and parenting: how to have them (if you want them), IVF (pray for my bank account) and what it's like to parent in a same-sex relationship.

I, like many indoctrinated people, used to believe a baby needed a mum and a dad. When I realised I wouldn't be able to provide that for my unborn child I felt a lot of shame. I might be gay, but my heart still melts when I see videos of a dad plaiting their daughter's hair or teaching them how to play baseball in the park. But maybe that's because we celebrate dads for doing the absolute bare minimum, while mums are balancing the load of everything else?

When I think about what my mum did compared to my dad, it baffles me. She worked full-time, raised three children, ferried us to whatever clubs and groups we had joined, regularly took me to auditions and work (we lived two hours out of London), walked two dogs, cooked dinners, arranged playdates, cleaned the house.

My dad went to work . . . and generally came home after we were in bed.

And somehow that's deemed a healthy parenting situation? Like men who refer to looking after their children as babysitting . . . you're not babysitting, it's your child – you're parenting! A lot of dads are absent and can do more damage by careering in and out of their child's life, so I rejigged my thinking of the whole 'a mum and dad are needed' scenario.

Society has taught us that if we don't have the 'traditional family unit' we are somehow unstable. The nuclear family was what we were taught to aspire to – and so now we must be letting our parents down (we're not). So as gay girlies, we have to redefine what a family looks like.

Going it alone

All a baby needs are people to really love it. Ideally two parents, but if not, just one. There are so many kickass single parents out there and that proves you don't need to be part of a double act. Just someone who can show different perspectives to a child, who can give it safety. Parents come in all different shapes and sizes, and no parents are perfect. When our kids turn seventeen, they are going to sit there blaming us for giving them trauma by not letting them do an exchange student programme in Singapore or buying them the wrong brand of trainers. I think if you go into parenting with that knowledge – that your job is to provide safety, guidance and love – you'll realise you can only do your best, and that some things are out of your hands.

I spent many a night praying my parents would get divorced, so they could remarry and I'd have some fun (not evil) step-parents. I was so jealous of other children who had four parents! I've often wondered if that's a universal thing, imagining different parenting scenarios. What would it be like being the kid of a lesbian couple? I spoke to my friend's children, a teenage brother and sister, Elsie and Tom, about the benefits (and few disadvantages) of having two mums! And I was warmed to the heart that it was a wholly positive conversation, one that showed how much love and respect they have for both their mums.

The consensus from them is that you can't miss what you've never had. Elsie says that from day one her mums were always open with her about the fact they don't know her dad, and on Father's Day, when her class were pritt-sticking cards for their dads, she'd just make one for her mum. Her friends grew up with her having two mums, so they've never made a big deal out of it. But Tom says he's definitely found male role models to help him along the way. He says he does have moments where he sees a dad and son on the street, or a nuclear family, and that sometimes he feels a pang of longing to experience that, even though his mums try to fill the roles that a dad might have played. Tom wants to live in a world where you don't have to battle the culture of trying to fit in v. the culture of being who you are, and is so proud of his mums living authentically.

Homophobia exists everywhere, but in 2025 the younger generations are much more fluid about their sexuality and there are openly queer couples throughout schools. It's not seen as a big thing any more. Prejudice is still rife in schools for all sorts of reasons, but being gay isn't the exclusive slur it was when I was young. Tom says that in arguments people occasionally weaponise the fact he has two mums and will throw out 'Your mum's gay' at him. His response: 'Your point being?' It's always been something he's embraced, and he does feel like he's more in tune with his emotions than his male peers.

Both Elsie and Tom did, however, agree that 'mother knows best' can be hard when you have two of them! Since mums are more emotionally in tune with their children, Elsie and Tom get a double dose of motherly instinct. They both admit this makes it hard to get away with anything they don't want their mums knowing about!

As for being a lesbian mum? In most ways it's the same as being any kind of mum.

You still have to make sure this little being is fed, changed and taken care of. Lisa is a mum of two girls with her partner Ciara, who had her first daughter the same time as her older sister. They were both trying to keep their tiny human alive and navigated the same things. Lisa found mother–baby groups a challenge when people assumed she was married to man, and that this stigma exemplified the main difference between her and her sister's experience. Even in the most accepting environments, you're still going to have to deal with people's judgements. But when Lisa talked to her sister, it became clear that her wife was better at getting up in the night with her than her sister's husband. She witnessed the workload being shared more equally than in her sister's relationship and found huge gratitude in her and her wife navigating the new baby terrain together.

Both Elsie and Tom know that when they turn eighteen they would like to find their biological dad and potential other siblings and family members. It used to be that donors got to choose whether they were contactable, but now it's a legal requirement in the UK. Not knowing where half of you comes from could lead to a lifelong quest for acceptance, so to give young people this knowledge and freedom seems like the most sensible thing to do. (And on the plus side, if your kids are badly behaved you can just blame it on some man you don't know!)

Many women advise that it's not a good idea to have a baby with your male best friend. And while it might seem like a neat movie plot, it can get messy. Many a situation has played out where they happily agree to jizz in a cup for you with no strings attached and then the second they meet the baby they're like 'Oh fuck, that's my child' and maybe want more involvement than you initially agreed.

Picking your sperm donor from a clinic is the norm, but that's not to say you can't choose someone you know. Whoever is not giving birth essentially has to go through the adoption process to register themselves as the child's mother. We're not at a place yet where two mothers are on birth certificates automatically. When I spoke to Emma, whose little boy was a year old at the time, she talked about how overwhelming it all seemed at first. There were so many different options to consider and different packages and price points, it felt more like organising a holiday than bringing a human into the world. She and her partner explored different clinics, some of which had open events to explain the process to potential parents. She read many articles and tried to speak to other women who'd been through this process, but found social media the best way to connect with other women going through the same journey. Emma and her partner decided to get sperm from a sperm bank, where they were shown profiles of potential donors, complete with photos of them when they were babies. She was aware how much each cycle of IVF cost and felt lucky she got pregnant on her second round. Once her little boy was a few days old they registered her partner as his mother too.

While hetero couples with kids are rarely asked how they conceived their children, queer couples are regularly faced with this invasion of privacy. When approaching having children as women together you have a few options to consider: adoption, surrogacy (where an egg is donated or you can use your own), IVF or artificial insemination. Artificial insemination involves placing sperm directly inside your or your partner's uterus using a catheter. The hope is that one of your eggs will be fertilised by the sperm.

The most regular route for women is IVF. Eggs are collected from your ovaries, fertilised with sperm in a lab, and then the strongest embryo is transferred back into your uterus where – hopefully – it will attach to the lining and allow a healthy pregnancy to develop.

If you both want to be involved in the process you can have what's known as reciprocal IVF. In this procedure, the eggs are taken from one partner's ovaries, fertilised with donor sperm, and then placed into the other partner's uterus. Both of you are physically involved in the process, with one partner donating their eggs and becoming the 'biological mother', while the other partner carries the baby and experiences the pregnancy as the 'birth mother'. This enables motherhood to be a shared experience right from conception.

While the NHS does offer IVF for lesbian couples, both AI and IVF are expensive and can cost up to £5,000 a cycle, which brings me on to a question I think about a lot . . . how do we navigate the world in a lesbian relationship when we're statistically less better off than our straight peers?

The gender pay gap is real

I've had the shocking realisation that if I want to be rich, I'm going to have to become THE MAN, if you will. It's now £5 a latte and I can't give up my coffees, as having a little walk around carrying a decaf soy latte is one of my only lasting pleasures in life and I'm hanging on by a thread here, guys. Is it financially viable to be a lesbian these days? Or the more imperative question: is it financially viable to be a woman? There are women CEOs kicking ass, running businesses and bringing in the dollar, but for most of society (as of 2024) women are still paid 7 per cent less than men for doing the same role according to the Office for National Statistics. And while we are working hard to close the gender pay gap, women are still, in effect, working for free from every November to the end of the year, every year.

For most of my life, my friend's mother had a mantra: 'Girls marry for money the first time, love the second.' She would say this while lounging languidly on the sofa, looking unbelievably glamorous. Teenage me was acutely aware she was on her first marriage . . . to my friend's dad. And while there's part of me that's inclined to find an eighty-year-old man to marry for the last few months of his life, I'm terrified he won't die and I'll be trapped like the girls in the Playboy mansion and I'll have to pull a *Saltburn* and then spend the rest of my life waiting for the cops to catch up with me and to be honest, my anxiety can't handle that. I assume I'm in trouble if someone just doesn't text me back.

No, we're going to have to find a way through this somehow.

We can be rich, successful and in love, and society will just have to take it . . . once I remember to pay my credit card bill . . .

Sexual Harassment of Working Women by Catharine A. MacKinnon is a brilliant book that looks at the intersection of women and economics. MacKinnon illustrates that under capitalism, women are segregated by gender and occupy a structurally inferior position in the workplace; this is hardly brand-new information, but she raises the question of why, even if capitalism 'requires some individuals to take low-status, low-paying positions why do those people have to be biologically female?'

MacKinnon cites a wealth of material documenting the fact that women are not only segregated in low-paying service jobs (as secretaries, domestics, nurses, typists, telephone operators, child-care workers, waitresses) but that the 'sexualisation of the woman' is part of the job. Central and intrinsic to the economic realities of women's lives is the requirement that women will 'market sexual attractiveness to men, who tend to hold the economic power and position to enforce their predilections'. For women in relationships with other women it means we'll potentially have to work harder to earn as much as our heterosexual peers. Can I give my future children the same financially stable life with two mums instead of a mum and a dad? So, there's still a glass ceiling to smash for all of womenkind and we're going to have to try to make ends meet until the tide starts turning. And no, I will not be giving up avocado.

19

What have you done today to make you feel proud?

Dear Diary,

I'm watching Billie Piper kiss Kaya Scodelario on a late-night BBC drama. I'm tucked into the corner of my parents' sofa. They're both asleep and I've snuck back down to watch it, having secretly recorded it on the telly. I must be about seventeen years old and this will be the first time I watch two women kiss on screen. When the moment happens, when their heads tilt and their bodies entwine, I rewind the moment, playing it back over and over again as if I'm trying to commit it to memory. Kaya Scodelario, in her school uniform looks like . . . well . . . me? It doesn't help she's getting off with Billie Piper and as Doctor Who's number one fan, I feel I could have written this scene in my mind. Until this point the only time I've seen a lesbian on screen is as the funny, slightly weird friend in the subplots of comedies. The token lesbian. And here is a representation of me, staring back at me.

In the sleepy suburbs of a Hampshire town it felt like lesbians barely existed. Bisexuality is something for your parents to tut at and say it's just a phase; we fear the responses to being gay, and if you don't date a boy who dresses in Hollister you may be exiled from the borough. But here in this moment, the real Rosie exists. This fantasy I've told no one, that I've been holding all alone, disappears. Maybe I'm not so weird after all?

I know that they're both straight actresses playing those roles, but in that moment it doesn't matter. I feel seen. I run up to bed and fall asleep knowing that maybe how I feel is OK. Maybe I too can date Billie Piper (let a girl dream, OK). Or maybe I can one day walk hand in hand down a windswept beach with someone I love.

As the years parade on, I wonder why there are so few British gay actresses. I can name a few from America (Sarah Paulson . . . what a queen!), but not many from England – and I know they must exist somewhere. As TV shows start commissioning series about the LGBTQIA+ community, I can't help but wish just sometimes there was an actual female, gay actor in the role. I didn't feel safe to come out as an actor. As a very straight-passing (what even is that?) girl, I was only ever cast as straight girls. Would I lose work? Would I lose my livelihood? What would happen if people found out? Perhaps if there had been actresses to look up to, I would have felt safe to do the same. And that is no hatred for our iconic Gentleman Jack. *Sometimes we need famous people to get shows made, and as there are very few lesbian actresses, the pool in which to cast from is quite small.*

If there had been representation, there's a high chance I wouldn't have buckled down, very solidly, on being straight. I wouldn't have spent a decade fitting a round peg into a square hole, and sometimes I feel I wouldn't have ended up in an abusive relationship with a man. The instinct to go with the status quo, not to risk my job, to live up to what society expected of me, was so strong. Sometimes I imagine a wonderful gay superwoman (played by Rebel Wilson, naturally) chasing me down an alleyway as I wander off to meet my soon-to-be boyfriend, scooping me up and flying off with me, shouting, 'GIRL FRIEND WE ARE NOT DOING THAT – WE ARE GOING TO FIND YOU A GIRLFRIEND.' If anyone wants to make a gay superhero movie please let me know. I'm available to write it. Maybe just a superhero who saves people from making lifelong mistakes and shows them they're actually gay. 'WAIT – YOU LIKE DR MARTENS AND DUNGAREES? I CAN HELP YOU! DON'T GO NEAR THAT MAN!' Marvel, call me.

Love,
Rosie x

Turns out I'm not the first person to think lesbians should be superheroes. The lesbian avengers exist. Yes, you read that right. Frustrated by society's erasure of lesbians, a group of women in nineties' New York fought back by creating the Lesbian Avengers, a group focused on issues vital to lesbian survival and visibility. Their campaigns had an electric theatricality: they ate fire, serenaded right-wing women outside churches, gave out chocolate in the street and handed out purple balloons to young people, branded 'Ask about lesbian lives'. Over time, the Lesbian Avengers grew into a national and international organisation, with groups across the world. The outsiders are the ones who get things done, who make changes, to society, to the world, to their lives. Now where's that movie? Don't worry – give me a couple of years, I'm making it.

As women who are part of the LGBTQIA+ community we slide into two minority categories, making our lives far from easy. This is the reason why activism is vital for our safety and happiness and to aid the lives of young women who follow us. I don't know about you, but I'm really not up for being killed for who I'm in love with. This isn't *The Hunger Games* (although Katniss Everdeen's spirit is something to carry with us while we fight the good fight). Women have been doing this on our behalf for years. The twentieth century saw a wave of organised activism to secure civil rights and freedoms for the LGBTQIA+ community, after a lifetime of hostility and legal prosecution. They fought for rights in employment, housing, military service and marriage. Then when the HIV/AIDs epidemic hit the world in the 1980s and made the lives of LGBTQIA+ people incredibly difficult, lesbians played a central role in shaping public health advocacy campaigns. Lesbians often took care of HIV patients when doctors or family members didn't want to. Throughout history, lesbians have been fighting for our rights. These women stood up for our future at a time when it was dangerous to do so.

So how do we stay empowered in the twenty-first century? We continue to fight. We find our tribe. Many LGBTQIA+ people find solace online; as I've already mentioned there are so many safe spaces on Instagram and TikTok to help you feel less alone. As a feminist, I still get a chill when I go to vote, remembering that women died for my right to do so. And it's the same for my right to live freely. For me, being a lesbian was informed entirely (like most things in society) by the patriarchy. Growing up, the male gaze made me believe that girls being gay was for men to get off to. The boys in the school cloakroom making jokes about girls kissing girls and huddling round their phones to watch porn . . . but then I'd hear them making homophobic comments to the students who actually were gay. So essentially, if I wanted to be celebrated by society as an out lesbian, I'd have to have my clothes off? And be making out with another girl? Otherwise I was weird? This is where representation comes in, and why it's so desperately important.

I just assumed I was going to be secretly miserable and in the closet for the rest of my life because I didn't have anyone to look up to. I didn't see a possibility for myself. Representation is hope. And hope is the strongest feeling there is. Give someone a sliver of hope and they can continue. But it's the isolation that's the killer. Living in silence, handling discrimination alone, feeling like you are an outsider. In recent years, so many of the movies that centre on the LGBTQIA+ experience have focused on or end in trauma. I don't need to point you in the direction of the most extreme version of that: *A Little Life*. The films usually follow the pattern of a person going on a journey to find love, and when they finally do, something terrible happens (cancer? car accident? take your pick) and one of them dies. I wanted LGBTQIA+ art that celebrates queer JOY! It's why shows such as *Heartstopper* are so vitally important. We can have very normal but equally pleasant lives too! Nothing dramatic has to happen! On the music scene, more and more artists are celebrating their queerness: Reneé Rap and Chappell Roan are flying the flag and their concerts are a safe hub for the queer community. Even most non-queer artists like Adele and Taylor Swift have made sure their spaces are safe and they are proud of their LGBTQIA+ audience members. And we can't forget the England World Champions, the Lionesses, who are not only changing the way people think about women's sport, but challenging people's ideas of what relationships look like.

Now with queer entertainment becoming more prevalent, we're giving little kids an idea of a future that can be whatever they'd like it to be. Nothing makes me happier than TikTok videos of tiny three-year-olds asking their aunts, 'Do you have a boyfriend? Or a girlfriend?' Children growing up knowing there's no difference. It's just the norm. And we're allowed to feel pride in ourselves.

Like many women, pride isn't something I feel easily. As women we've been conditioned to shrink and not take up space. Being outwardly anything gave me the message I was 'too much'. Women seen as being too big for their boots are vilified by the masses. Women are constantly self-deprecating, minimising, finding ways to celebrate other people so as to draw attention away from themselves. There's such a difference between showing up and being celebrated and being some egotistical drama queen. And yet we can't even do the former. But pride is vital to our survival. When people ask why Pride needs a month, I reply, 'Because there are people out there who believe they're better off dead than living as themselves.' It usually shuts them up pretty fast.

The first-ever Pride march was held exactly one year after the Stonewall riots, on 28 June 1970 in New York City. The

Stonewall uprising took place at the Stonewall Inn, after it was raided by the police in the early hours. Three nights of protest followed, with the LGBTQIA+ community, long frustrated by police brutality, finally fighting back. And lesbians were some of the key people involved in the act of resistance.

Pride became a day of honour for the impactful Stonewall uprising and eventually morphed into a whole month of recognition and celebration for the queer community. However, research by LGBT+ young people's charity Just Like Us suggests that only a third of schools celebrate Pride, LGBTQIA+ History Month or School Diversity Week, with 35 per cent of pupils and 38 per cent of teachers surveyed reporting school celebrations.

But we don't need to wait for June every year to feel proud of ourselves. It's something we can practise every day in order to live a happier life, with a whole load of self-compassion for ourselves.

When we start to have empathy for ourselves and for others – we become more connected to ourselves. When we can acknowledge the commonality of the human condition, that we're all who we are, something beautiful happens: we diminish the subtle pain of indifference. When we find self-compassion we tend to experience greater happiness and better relationships, which helps us move into connection with others. And at a time when more women than ever are exploring their sexuality, that's something we're after, right? That's why you've read this book? And as they say in *Derry Girls,* 'You can't move for lesbians. It's wall-to-wall lesbians out there.' It could be time for you to put it into practice.

A gay girl's manifesto

1   May you surround yourself with people who want the best for you.

2   May you remember that the people who truly love you for who you are will stick around.

3   May you keep safe in your mind, body, pleasure and day-to-day life.

4   May you remember you don't have to like rainbows.

5   May you buy a good pair of boots to kick homophobes with.

6   May you try not to fall in love with every older woman who shows you affection.

7   May you acquire a cat or other small animal to care for.

8   May you know that your sexuality can be the least interesting or most interesting thing about you - if that's what you wish.

9   May you know it's neither your job nor your responsibility to educate others on the LGBTQIA+ community.

10 May you remember you don't have to get that tattoo.

11 May you be kind to others and most importantly, yourself.

12 May we accept ourselves exactly as we are in this moment.

Epilogue

Sometimes I imagine myself at forty-five.

For a long time I really didn't think I was going to live that long. I was convinced I was going to be killed off by thirty in a bike accident . . . and there was that one time the toaster ended up precariously close to the bath . . .

It's Friday night. I have finally got my style sorted (thank God, she can pull off that trench coat now), it's raining and I fall through the door of my north London house with a clatter of book bags and bicycles. I've just picked my daughter up from ballet. She marches down the hallway in her frog wellies and yellow rain mac, tutu poking through, her little legs splashed with mud. We're going to have beans on toast and a bubble bath while we wait for Mummy to get home. My wife works in . . . Finance? Hopefully? Unless my career as a writer has really taken off, in which case maybe she teaches at the local primary school? When she arrives home we share dessert on our much-loved red velvet sofa and watch our favourite TV series until we fall asleep.

The next morning, I wake and pad down to the kitchen, no doubt to an angry cat weaving its way around my ankles, meowing for breakfast. No one's up yet. It's still outside. I make coffee and turn on the radio. There's something familiar in the static that I used to use to drown out the noise in my head. . . the noise that's not there any more. The trees are turning for winter. I am now a home to someone. I'm almost afraid of the saturation of this contentment. Just me and my little life. I grab the paper on our doormat that reads, 'We hope you like cats', and run back up the stairs to bed, the chilly morning air brushing my thighs. Our daughter (Summer? Willow?) launches herself on to our duvet and we cuddle for a while. Later we'll join friends for a walk on Hampstead Heath before having lunch in the pub.

There will be a moment (maybe when I climb the heath in momentous fashion looking out over the rolling city, or when I'm immersed in my standalone bathtub, or when I'm rushing to the school gates to pick up my daughter) . . .

Where I'll wonder how I got here.

How I'm not alone any more.

How I managed to create the life I longed for.

With tiny unnoticeable steps in the right direction. The jigsaw puzzle pieces that for so long felt muddled and creased. Each fragment of pain, joy, terror and hope slotted together to make a very ordinary, extraordinary life.

My only wish is the same for you.

Acknowledgements

The idea for this book took shape over dinner with my partner-in-crime, who also happens to be my agent, Anna Dixon (and her wonderful husband, Alex, who feeds our ideas). Thank you for your endless support, hard work and cheerleading which have changed my life.

Thank you to Bernadette Marron, my brilliant editor for her expertise, skill and fighting the good fight – and to Sarah Thomas and everyone at Piatkus. This book was nothing but a joy to create. I am so lucky.

To everyone who generously lent their time, life experience and expertise – the biggest thank you. It wouldn't have been possible without you all. Especially Ellen Jones, Lolly Issacs and Jessica Revell – the women who have shown me what's possible.

Thank you to Amber and Kate for podcast-length voice notes, brilliant friendship and making sure I have the space to write. And Katy, for always being by my side.

And lastly to Vix, the brightest woman I know. Thank you.